Thinking about patients

Thinking about patients

David Misselbrook MSc, FRCGP, DRCOG

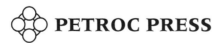 PETROC PRESS

Petroc Press, an imprint of LibraPharm Limited

Distributors
Plymbridge Distributors Limited, Plymbridge House, Estover Road, Plymouth PL6 7PZ, UK

Published in the United Kingdom by
LibraPharm Limited
Gemini House
162 Craven Road
NEWBURY
Berkshire
RG14 5NR
UK

A catalogue record for this book is available from the British Library

ISBN 1 900603 49 7

Typeset by WordSpace, Lewes, East Sussex
Printed and bound in the United Kingdom by Bell & Bain, Glasgow G46 7UQ

Contents

Dedication

To Ruth

Song of Songs, Ch 4 v 7

Preface:
How to use this book

This book was written to promote a multidimensional model of medicine. The whole book puts this model into context, but you may not want the whole package.

If you want to take a step back and consider the changing role of medicine in society, then read Chapters 1–4 and Chapter 10. If you are interested solely in learning about a multidimensional medical model, then read Chapters 5–10. But who knows – you may even enjoy the book as a whole!

You may find that that you want to learn more as part of your own Professional Development Plan. The references and literature reviews will give you an excellent start to further study. Or you may just want to use this book as a reference work for the social science literature – the index and chapter headings will help you find what you need.

Chapter 1 explores the scope, achievements and problems of medicine at the beginning of the 21st century.

Chapter 2 explores the doctor's model of disease and contrasts it with the patient's model of illness.

Chapter 3 explores how the doctor's model is generated by the particular and extraordinary world that the doctor inhabits, and how that world is constructed.

Chapter 4 explores how the world that the patient inhabits is different from the doctor's world.

Chapters 5–9 describe and explore the non-biomedical elements of a multidimensional medical model. They describe how disease, illness and medicine can only be properly understood by including our individual thoughts and our social and cultural programming as part of the whole picture.

Chapter 10 poses some questions relevant to the ongoing debate about the role and the future of medicine.

I hope that what you choose to read will make you think. Above all I hope it will help you to think about the needs of patients.

April 2001   DM

All patients' names, demographic details and many medical details have been changed in order to preserve confidentiality.

Acknowledgements

There is nothing new under the sun ... Of making many books there is no end
Attributed to Solomon. Ecclesiastes Ch 1 v 9, Ch 12 v 12

I have learned that books are not written in a vacuum. This book grew out of my professional life and reflection, and in this I owe a debt to many.

What concern I have for patients started with my parents' example of care for others tempered by thoughtful understanding, and their similar encouragement and nurturing of my own development.

I owe much to my own professional mentors, especially Manny Tuckman my trainer, and Roger May who enabled me to move towards a reflective professional life. Alan Ruben and Budgie Savage have helped me to grow, and have shown me how to help other learners.

The UMDS (now GKT) MSc helped clarify and develop much of my thinking. I benefited from the ideas and animated discussion of the other members of "MSc 10". I gained much from all the MSc tutors, especially David Armstrong, Nikki Britten and Jane Ogden.

David Armstrong and Martin Edwards kindly read the first drafts of this book, and their feedback has improved it greatly. Peter Clarke from Petroc has been amazingly encouraging, and patient with the time it has taken me to complete the project.

I am grateful to my partners, Nicholas Surridge, David Sharpe and Janet McCredie, for allowing me to take a sabbatical to do the research for the book, and bearing with me as I wrote it. I am grateful to Abdol Tavabie for helping me to obtain funding for the sabbatical, and for his interest in the book. Henry Tegner, my co-course organiser on the Lewisham GP vocational training scheme has been generous with his friendship and support.

Above all I am fortunate to have the acceptance and support of Ruth, my wife, and the encouragement of three fantastic children, Clare, Tom and Jamie, who make life great.

Foreword by
Dr Roger Neighbour

As I write, Tony Blair's government has just been returned for a second term, by what – despite being supported by only a minority of the lowest turnout for a generation – it is pleased to call a "landslide". We doctors should no doubt rejoice that improving the public services, and especially the NHS, heads the list of the new administration's promises. That joy, however, may be tempered with a heart-sinking "here we go again" realisation that "improving" is synonymous in the political lexicon with "driving through reform". Whether or not reform is what is needed rather than man-power and money, and whether or not "driving through" is the best way of achieving it, it looks as if we are in for an extension of what David Misselbrook in his closing chapter describes as a "decade of un-navigated change".

Also as I write, and far from coincidentally, the BMA at its annual conference is wondering what can be done about plummeting morale amongst the nation's GPs, as evidenced by another recent landslide vote to threaten resignation if more realism and common sense cannot be incorporated into our terms of service. To a profession now genuinely sensitised to the merits of patient-centredness in our consultations, the frustration, resentment and impotence at finding ourselves on the receiving end of a top-down imposed political agenda is particularly painful. Most will be thinking it, some will be muttering it under their breath, a few will try to shout it loud enough for the nation to hear – "They just don't understand!"

Well, what is it that "they" don't understand? Everything that's in this book, for a start: that general practice is where science wears its human face; that general practice is the natural home of today's "Renaissance man"; that in general practice the notion that technical advance equates to social advance is plainly revealed for a fallacy; and that to a general practitioner it is no paradox to know that the bottom line is seldom the bottom line.

History reverberates with examples, many more momentous than our own, of how people might act in defence of their core values when they find themselves out of temper with the prevailing political or cultural climate. When Henry VIII dissolved the monasteries the Catholic priests went underground, and established a network of supporters happy to help keep the tradition alive until more liberal times returned. As National Socialism infected Germany between the wars, decent citizens who tried to conceal their beliefs by marching in step with false smiles often found camouflage to be an insecure refuge. Others, inclined like Captain Kidd to bury their treasure on some remote island, should take heed that, if the map is too vague or the search too arduous, the gold may be lost for ever.

So what is a GP to do, torn between the imperatives, on the one hand, to provide patients with the best in biomedical advances as effectively and equitably as possible, and, on the other, to insist that the solutions to human problems that are complex and long-standing in their origin are unlikely to be as quick and simple as political convenience would wish?

In general we must be humble enough to take criticism and embrace constructive change, yet at the same time brave enough to guard our treasure from harm. The treasure of general practice is the richness of its philosophical underpinning, the eclectic nature of its academic origins, the breadth of thought needed to comprehend every patient who walks through the consulting room door, the sheer quizzical scepticism with which it eyes every attempt to reduce health care to something one-dimensional and neatly quantifiable.

Guarding this kind of treasure means, today, communicating it. It means writing it down, comprehensively and persuasively. It means getting it published, read, appreciated. That is David Misselbrook's achievement. He is an erudite and thoughtful doctor, a true polymath, a man with a commanding view of the big picture, and yet at the same time someone clearly in love with the fine detail of professional life, the greater and lesser human comedies and tragedies with which general practice abounds. If every aspiring and practising GP would read his book, and maybe the odd bureaucrat and politician too – well, who knows? Maybe they will understand.

Roger Neighbour
GP, Abbots Langley, Hertfordshire
Author of *The Inner Consultation* and *The Inner Apprentice*
Convenor, Panel of MRCGP Examiners, 1997–2002

 # Introduction

> *Every physician must be rich in knowledge, and not only of that which is written in books; his patients should be his book, they will never mislead him.*
>
> Paracelsus, The Book of Tartaric Diseases

> *When all possible questions of science are answered, the problems of life remain unanswered.*
>
> Ludwig Wittgenstein

Chapter summary

Medicine is practised within a social context that co-determines its aims and methods. Areas of "social progress" have undergone radical re-evaluation in the last two decades. A similar re-evaluation of medicine is needed. Our use of evidence-based medicine is too narrow in the type of evidence that is admissible.

Progress

The problem of progress

I remember progress. Science would solve the problems of the world. The cities would be rebuilt as fast as we could pour concrete. There were these walkways between the blocks of flats – one day you would be able to stroll from the Thames right through South London without crossing the street. As housing changed people too would change, living together in bold new communities free from the squalor and ignorance of yesterday. Farming was becoming scientific too. Out with the hedgerows, on with the fertiliser. The whole world was joining in. In Amazonia there were fearless new cities where once there was only useless rain forest. Wildlife and whales beware. This is the modern age.

Actually most of this passed me by. I grew up in a sleepy rural town where they didn't have the 1960s. They weren't quite sure whether news of Queen Victoria's death mightn't be a malicious rumour. I remember my excitement as I escaped the backwaters of my childhood and went to Medical School. London. One great leap and I was part of the modern world. But the modern world seemed to be changing. Whales good, concrete bad. Rainforest good, concrete still bad. Progress changed.

Medical progress?

Perhaps medicine is now in its version of that awkward cultural period of the early 1970s. Somewhere just between the Beatles and Abba. We know something is being lost, but the world moves on. In the explosion of "progress" after the War society made many mistakes. Wall-to-wall concrete wasn't such a good idea. Billions of pounds are now being spent in ripping it up. Maybe hedgerows and whales were worth keeping after all. We have to stop the bus and go back for them. Does this mean we are returning to the past? To a lost world of slums and cider with Rosie? No. We are finding new ways. The new housing in the borough where I work looks very similar to our Victorian heritage, but with better plumbing and insulation. We can have the best of both worlds if we try.

So, what of "modern" medicine? If anything it is a victim of its own success. As a boy in the 1960s Dr Kildare taught me that technology was the key. If we were smart enough we could fix anything. Medicine's hall of fame has had a powerful effect on our culture. Antibiotics, angiography, A&E, appendectomy, AZT, antidepressants, anti-ulcer drugs. I won't bore you with B–Z. HG Wells would have given his right arm to be shown round my surgery, never mind a teaching hospital. But could Western medicine have turned out differently?

Medicine doesn't happen in a vacuum

Western medicine is a powerful system. It shows us a way of looking at illness, and a way of intervening. But it is not the only approach to illness. Western medicine works as it does because it relates to other aspects of Western living. Like any cultural system it is not written in stone. It could be done differently. And how it is done only makes sense in the context of the rest of our culture.

Our medicine has become more and more about fixing things. Fixing things that go wrong, and fixing the risk of things going wrong. But if we are to look at the interaction of medicine with people we must take a step back. We must ask what things should be fixed, and what seen as normal. We will recognise that such questions can only make sense when seen in their cultural setting. We cannot extricate the things we do as doctors from the lives of the people we do them to. Both our patients and ourselves are part of a changing world.

We must also ask who should be giving the answers. How can we as doctors, as experts, negotiate with autonomous patients about aims and motives in medicine?

This book examines the way Western medicine affects peoples' lives, and the way our culture – the sum of all our lives – affects medicine. If medicine and culture affect one another then you can't understand medicine without thinking about that interaction.

What sort of progress?

The brutal and de-humanising architecture of the mid-twentieth century was produced as a result of magnificent theories. Le Corbusier famously defined buildings as "machines designed for living in". But there was just one thing wrong with "modern movement" homes. People don't want to live in them. I want my home to be human in its references. I want it to reflect my own personal eccentricities and my own cultural background. I want it to be homely. And I don't want the roof to leak inconsolably after ten years.

The key to our change in attitudes in the 1970s and 1980s was the realisation that the model of "progress" we had was too narrow, too selective of what could be admitted as evidence, too enticing in its hygienic glossiness. Too simple-minded. So it wasn't the idea of a "machine for living in" that was wrong, it was the modernists' inadequate model of "living".

So how does this apply to medicine? I am not suggesting that we should lessen the value we place on evidence. No return to Rousseau's "noble savage". When my appendix swells I want it taken out as fast as the next man does. No. The key is to widen the scope of evidence we use to guide health care – more evidence, not less.

We are supposed to make our diagnoses in the physical, psychological and social dimensions. If this is really our belief, then let us demand evidence from these dimensions.

My problem with current evidence-based medicine (EBM) is that it works like this:

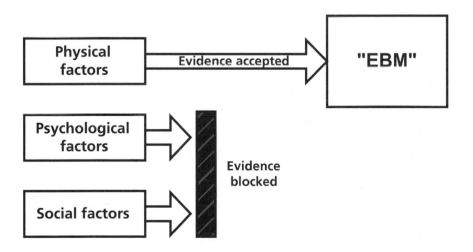

My model for "Real EBM" (REBM?) would be like this:

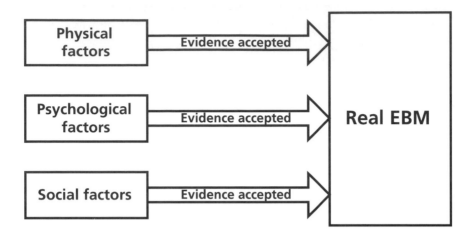

The problem with this model of course is that in including physical, psychological and social factors we are not mixing like with like. How do you compare one life saved with an indeterminate amount of anxiety in thousands of women having smears?

This objection marginalises both human judgement and patient autonomy. If taking into account non-comparable variables is not a doctor's core job then what is? I don't believe that we should let our job be whittled away to that of a technician just to satisfy the control hunger of managers and politicians.

The problem with EBM is that it is simplistic. It can only work by restricting our gaze in the search for evidence. Having restricted our evidence to the biomedical we then restrict our analysis and our guidelines to this model also. And of course once we've got a guideline then we don't need to think.

This book is a campaign for "real evidence-based medicine". Let's take off the blinkers and stop pouring the concrete. Medicine without an understanding of human values is not only banal but inhumane.

During the 1970s and 1980s there was a real attempt to become more patient-oriented, spurred on by the work of writers such as Byrne and Long,[1] Pendleton,[2] Tuckett[3] and Neighbour.[4] The 1990s have seen us overtaken by issues of funding and organisation. The challenge of patient-centred practice is not a box we can tick and leave behind. The need to be patient-centred has been well stated, but what this means is still largely uncharted.

Constructing patient-centred medicine first entails deconstructing the world of medicine and the world of the patient in order to redefine the relationship between them. This is the aim of this book.

References

1 Byrne L and Long B. Doctors talking to patients. London: RCGP Publications, 1976.
2 Pendleton D, Schofield T, Tate P and Havelock P. The Consultation: an approach to learning and teaching. Oxford: Oxford University Press, 1984.
3 Tuckett D et al. Meetings between experts. London: Tavistock Publications, 1985.
4 Neighbour R. The Inner Consultation. Lancaster: MTP Press, 1987.

1 The biomedical model

Gold that buys health can never be ill spent.

John Webster and Thomas Dekker (c. 1580–c. 1625;
c. 1572–c. 1632)
Westward Ho!

Apollo was held the god of physic and sender of disease.
Both were originally the same trade, and still continue.

Jonathan Swift
Thoughts on Various Subjects, Moral and Diverting

Chapter summary

Biomedicine has been a huge success within Western culture. It can fix medical problems that have never previously been treatable and that cannot be fixed by other medical systems. The greatest advances have occurred over recent decades when the intellectual basis of science is seen as less secure than before, emphasising medicine's reliance upon technology rather than science per se.

There are however increasingly widely recognised limits to the success of biomedicine. This has led to a reaction against the biomedical model, and concerns for its problematisation of normality. Another problem is what the biomedical model leaves out. Our current biomedical system is vulnerable to hijack, and there is uncertainty as to who will win the current battle for its control.

In this book I will be criticising many aspects of modern medicine. It seems only fair therefore to start with a report of its successes.

The triumph of biomedicine

An everyday medical triumph

When I was seven I fought in the street with an older boy who concluded our battle by forcefully pushing me backwards. My right upper arm caught on the metal hasp in the pillar of the front gate. It felt funny, so I conceded defeat and ran indoors. I took off my shirt and was scared to see a deep wound with a large skin flap hanging open. Breaking the childhood code of silence, I showed Mum. I suddenly got a lot of attention. I was wrapped in a blanket, and Dad was summoned from the depths of his study to take me to the Casualty Department of Kettering Hospital. The deep muscular tear required reconstruction under a general anaesthetic. I emerged with an impressive number of stitches and an even more impressive triangular sling. Bewildering quantities of sweets appeared.

The muscular injury didn't get infected, and my arm works fine. Two outcomes that we take for granted, but a result that in previous generations would have been possible only with extreme good luck. Kettering Hospital provided me with something that worked better than good luck, and its about time that I said a public thank you. A small triumph perhaps, but important to me and to my family. The kind of small triumph that is repeated thousands of times a day around the country, and which is the reason we pay for a health service.

Medicine works

The phenomenon of Western biomedicine is huge. It consumes about 6% of GDP in the UK, currently about £44billion per year.[1] You and I spend £750 per capita in tax every year on the NHS. Before the 1990 reforms split the NHS into smaller units, the NHS was the biggest employer in Europe after the Red Army. In England in 1998–9 there were 11,984,000 finished consultant episodes, 12,811,000 attendances at A&E Departments,[2] and 17,369,000 Community Health Worker contacts.[3] There were 251,000,000 GP consultations in 1998-9.[4] The NHS is one of the few organisations still bigger than Microsoft. In other Western countries the story is the same or greater. The USA spent 7.4% of GDP on health care in 1970. By 1997 this had risen to 14.2%.[5]

How did medicine get so big? Partly because it works.

It's easy to forget what we owe to Western medicine. If I suffered an open compound lower limb fracture today I would expect to be scooped up by paramedics, given effective analgesia in A&E, and treated rapidly by a trained Orthopaedic surgeon with internal fixation of the fracture. I would hobble out of hospital in one piece, and be walking again with near-zero disability within a few months.

Four hundred years ago my fate would have been to lie in agony being cared for by my relatives until I died of septicaemia from a wound infection or pressure sores. Two hundred years ago my fate would have been a cart ride to a surgeon who would have amputated my leg without anaesthetic. I would then have a 50/50 choice between death from infection or permanent disability and crutches.

Consider the following list of common conditions:

- dropsy/heart failure
- diabetes mellitus
- septicaemia

- obstructed labour
- schizophrenia
- advanced cataracts
- advanced osteoarthritis of the hip
- bowel obstruction.

If you were affected by one of these, would you choose a medieval treatment system or modern medicine? Consider what it means to be a patient faced with any of these diseases, and the appalling suffering that was inevitable in the past but that can be fixed now. There are also public health triumphs such as the eradication of smallpox, immunisation, sanitation, antimalarials, and preventative medicine. It is no wonder that Roy Porter, quoting from Samuel Johnson, entitles his history of medicine "The greatest benefit to mankind."[6]

How Western medicine happened

Western medicine is often dated back to Hippocrates in the 4th century BC. He was the first Western thinker to formulate diseases as natural processes that are open to rational study. Without this idea doctors were confined to the world of superstition. In this sense therefore it is fair to view Hippocrates as the father of Western medicine.

As well as taking this giant step for mankind, Hippocrates is also famous for the first code of medical ethics. It would be good if biomedical and ethical progress were always bound so closely together.

Between Hippocrates and Vesalius in the 16th century AD there was a gradual growth of teaching on health and disease, based on little science beyond Aristotle. Notable figures such as Galen and Paracelsus formulated the ideas of their day. These were then transmitted from teacher to pupil within a theory of knowledge based on authority rather than experiment. Underlying theories related to the current cosmological and alchemical models. The Basic Medical Sciences syllabus of the day would consist of subjects such as humoral theory and astrology. As in any age the role and the models of medicine could only be understood within the worldview and culture of the day.

Vesalius managed to be around at the right moment to be credited with a change of gear in Western medicine. He was a fiery radical with the apparently absurd idea that direct observation is a more important source of knowledge than the authority of ancient great men passed on through a long chain of teachers. It is easy for us to mock the idea of authority as the main source of knowledge. But what if we remove from our world the comfort of computerised scanning equipment, research laboratories and peer review journals? If you will humour my dubious historical method for a moment we could begin to imagine a different sort of argument (and you get extra marks if you spot the Brecht quotation):

Prof X: So Vesalius, what is this new idea of yours, a "research grant"?

Vesalius: It's a really exciting development, sir. If the University will fund me then I can perform a series of anatomies and make detailed observations on what I actually see. We would not have to rely on centuries-old knowledge alone. New observations may be more accurate, and we may make new advances. Who knows where it may lead? I see a Nobel Prize beckoning.

Prof X: Good heavens man! Were you born yesterday? Don't you know that knowledge is based on reason, not on fallible observation? Galen has stood the test of time. His teachings have been proven as the greatest gift to mankind for more than a millennium. Think how reliable they must be to stand up to such a test. Why on earth should we open ourselves up to new realms of inaccuracy when the research has already been done? Why should we replace secure knowledge with fashionable whim? Are we to establish human society on doubt, and no longer on belief? And your suggestion is impudent. I am a Professor here because I am part of a precious chain of knowledge that has been passed on from Galen, from Aristotle, from Hippocrates himself. What of the publishing houses who devotedly copy their works, bringing out a revised edition every century or so? How can they possibly publish a new work only to be told you want it updated after a mere decade or two? You expect me to give you a research grant so that ten minutes later you can tell me I am wrong and that you know better? You'll be after my editorship of the PMJ [Padua Medical Journal] next. I think not!

The opposition to new ideas was (as ever) entirely reasonable within its cultural and epistemological setting. Despite this, Vesalius was one of the pioneers who broke the mould of authority and started to shape a new mould of empirical experimentation. The human body and the processes within it gradually came to be seen as open to rational analysis and modelling. They were not simply inscrutable and unchangeable essential properties of man, but consisted of mechanisms that could be unravelled.

It is easy to fail to see how the body could appear so inscrutable that we should feel that the only policy is to rely on static authority for our therapeutic interventions. We can enjoy the arrogance of retrospect. Perhaps a modern analogy would be our understanding of the essential nature of subatomic particles. Sure, we're discovering new ones every day, and we know ever more about what they do. But we know nothing at all about why they do what they do. Matter attracts antimatter just because it does. $E=mc^2$ – because it does. I know how many unstable atoms will decay over a given period of time but I have no model at all to tell me which ones. I know not if Schrödinger's cat lives. All these things to us are just the way things are. At the moment they are the inseparable properties or essence of the things themselves.

Imagine that every function and malfunction of the body is simply its inherent and inscrutable essential property, albeit open to the external influences of the stars and the fates, and you will begin to understand what it was to be a pre-enlightenment doctor. It doesn't make you irrational or daft, it just leaves you doing the best you can within a complex and consistent but largely impotent model.

The key, then, to the success of biomedicine is the experimental, empirical view it takes of the body. This started with the discipline of Anatomy, but led on with advances in 18th- and 19th-century chemistry to physiology. Microscopy led on to cell biology, biochemistry led on to pharmacology. Gradually the basic medical sciences took over from the ancient humoral and astrological models of illness.

Most significantly of all, post mortem studies led to the concept of illness being caused by distinct disease entities. This was a revolution. Previously all one had to do would be to describe a symptom. A flux (diarrhoea) or a chill (fever) would be accepted as diagnostic terms. Now they become symptoms, requiring a diagnosis in pathological terms. The treatment would previously be aimed at the symptom, or at the whole body disturbance that the symptom implied. Now treatment must be aimed at the disease entity causing the symptom. Disease was for the first time separated from illness. It is in the study of disease that biomedicine grew as an intellectually distinct Western entity. It is the study of disease that has won biomedicine its glittering success.

It would be easy to see the gradual rise of modern biomedicine as an inevitable triumph from this point on. Strangely enough this is not so. By the beginning of the 19th century there would be relatively few treatments that would be much superior to those given by a mediaeval practitioner, although the science base had progressed through the 17th and 18th centuries. By the end of the 19th century the foundations of modern surgery, anaesthesia and antisepsis were in place. However, non-surgical treatments were only beginning the very earliest stages of the explosive growth curve that we have seen in the 20th century.

Medicine uses technology more than it does science. There is usually a latent period between fundamental scientific discoveries and their use in medicine. Remember that Cochrane's famous monograph calling for randomised controlled trials (RCTs) to be the arbiter of therapeutic efficacy was published not in 1872 but in 1972.[7]

A very brief history of medicine

Consider how rapidly the pace of progress in the West has accelerated:

Pre-Renaissance: Traditional use of medicinal plants, midwifery, simple bonesetting.
   Available drugs: alcohol, morphine.
1500–1850: Gradual improvement in surgical treatment of trauma.

New drugs: digitalis, citrus fruit.

Late 1800s: Anaesthesia, antisepsis, hygiene, public health and sanitation, germ theory, X-rays, classification of mental illness.

New drugs: Chloral, thyroxine, quinine, aspirin.

1900–1950: Psychotherapy, routine major surgery, ECT.

New drugs: Paracetamol, barbiturates, salvarsan, insulin, penicillin, lithium.

1950s: Smoking identified as a cause of cancer, DNA structure discovered, early ultrasound.

New drugs: Tricyclics, steroids, β-blockers, diuretics, anti-tuberculars.

1960s: Organ transplantation, CPR, Cardiac surgery, immunisation.

New drugs: Benzodiazepines, antipsychotics, new antibiotics, oral contraception, chemotherapy.

1970s: CT scanning, test tube babies, monoclonal antibodies, supremacy of RCTs, endoscopy.

New drugs: H_2 antagonists, asthma inhalers, NSAIDs.

1980s: Eradication of smallpox.

New drugs: Aciclovir, ACE inhibitors

1990s: Experimental gene therapy, MRI scanning.

New drugs: Prozac, anti-*helicobacter* therapy, Viagra.

Biomedicine triumphant

The speed of progress is dizzying. Hertzler (as quoted by Porter), reviewing medical practice over the first half of the 20th century, said "I can scarcely think of a single disease that the doctors actually cured during those early years". All that doctors could do was "to relieve suffering, set bones, sew up cuts and open boils on small boys".[8] Within a single generation the panoply of investigation and cure available to us increased at an explosive pace. Within a generation the biomedical project to cure or contain all disease seemed to be well underway.

The success of biomedicine can be viewed from two perspectives. First, it has achieved great success as the dominant cultural response to disease. If a passer-by experiences severe central chest pain, will I sit him down with a nice cup of tea or will I dial 999? Biomedicine is overwhelmingly seen as the normative response to any serious threat to health. Our surgeries and hospitals have never been so full. The medical sections at our bookshops never so well stocked. Our carrier bags from Boots never so bulging. The costs alone demonstrate that biomedicine is a huge commercial and cultural success.

But what about the more important measure of success? Do we make people better? Does biomedicine work? This is a far harder question to answer than one might think. It was scarcely a question at all until the 1970s. In 1949 Lord Horder asked "Whither medicine?", to which his answer was "Why, whither else but straight ahead".[9] The post-war explosion of biomedical fixes has been an exhilarating ride for those on board. It is self-evident to us as doctors that we do sometimes save lives, and often give effective treatments that reduce morbidity.

The counterblast of the 1970s was first trumpeted by Ivan Illich in his controversial classic *Medical Nemesis*, published in 1976.[10] This placed the downside to Western medicine at centre stage. There have been many attempts to determine whether medicine is overall of benefit or disbenefit to patients.[11,12,13,14] Recent opinion tends to the view that biomedicine does have an overall positive impact on our health, but that the degree of benefit is difficult to measure. One contribution to this problem by Bunker is worth review:

Literature review

Bunker J, 1995. Medicine matters after all. Journal of the Royal College of Physicians of London, 29, No 2: 105–12.

Bunker has made a brave attempt to quantify the benefits in morbidity and mortality from current Western medical practice. He does not quote comparative outcome measures. His mortality figures are derived from the decline in death rates in a few major conditions where RCTs and meta-analyses are able to give a measure of the degree of benefit from medical intervention. Morbidity figures are similarly calculated from RCT data of benefit, together with the average duration of illness.

Bunker concludes that three of the seven years of increase in life expectancy since 1950 can be attributed to medical care. He estimates that medical care provides on average five years of partial relief from the deterioration in quality of life associated with chronic disease.

Unfortunately any bold attempt to put figures on overall medical benefit is bound to rely on a whole series of assumptions which must work together for the model to be valid. It is easy to drive a hearse through Bunker's science. (Do RCTs reflect treatment outcomes in the real world? What about his selection of evidence? Where are the real outcome figures? What about iatrogenic illness?)

This paper is therefore a bold but vulnerable attempt to answer a question of burning importance. If we believe the paper then it provides us with some of the best evidence we have for a belief in the value of Western medicine.

Bunker's views are wide open to challenge, but what alternative to such figures can we have? Scientifically robust figures could only be obtained by randomly allocating a whole population to Western medical care or no biomedical care status. Such a study might have difficulty obtaining ethical committee approval. If Bunker is right in saying that my £750 per annum in tax buys me three years of extra life and five years of partial relief from suffering and disability, then I say it's money well spent.

It is reasonable to see biomedicine as one of the great triumphs of the West: a huge success as a business enterprise, and truly the "greatest benefit to mankind", even if Johnson was somewhat premature with his accolade.

Problems with biomedicine

Unfortunately we cannot leave matters there. Medicine may have won glittering prizes, but not everyone is applauding. Since the 1950s there has been increasing criticism of Western medicine from Sociologists. From the 1970s politicians and patients have joined in. So what's wrong with biomedicine? Alongside the success there is the dark side to biomedicine, which we prefer to keep locked in the attic. There are a number of issues:

- The limitations of the scientific foundations of medicine
- The limits of biomedicine's success
- Iatrogenic problems
- What biomedicine leaves out
- Functional illness
- The problematisation of normality
- Biomedicine's vulnerability to hijack.

The rest of the chapter briefly examines these problems.

Problems with science

Medicine's most spectacular successes have occurred over the last fifty years. It is perhaps ironic that over this same period science, medicine's greatest patron, has changed from an all-conquering monolithic superhero to a self-doubting adolescent ever seeking the next makeover. (An excellent summary of this transformation has been written by Chalmers – it is well worth reading.[15])

Inductivism was the basis of science in the last century. Inductivism views the world as a large, complex but concrete machine. Rather like a big jigsaw. We can examine lots of bits of the machine and see how they work together in order to induce universal laws about the whole system, even though we know we will never have the time to look at every piece individually. X has always happened, therefore X must always happen. True, Hume had pointed out the logical fallacy of this in the 18th century, but this could be conveniently forgotten. What did old philosophers know of science?

In the 20th century Bertrand Russell restated the objections to this approach with his inductivist turkey which "proved" by careful and repeated observation that at 9 am he is always fed, only to have his theory tragically refuted on Christmas Eve. Some have sought to preserve the usefulness of inductivism by limiting its claims to notions of probability. Inductivism is still the basis of the "popular" view of science. It is a useful method because it is common sense and often works.

In the last half-century philosophy has got even. The philosophers of science produced a number of arguments that could no longer be ignored. These swept away the cosy monolithic 19th-century view of science as an absolute repository of truth.

Observation is theory-dependent

All science is based upon observation. But we do not observe the world in a passive way. Twentieth-century psychology has taught us we are active participants in the act of perception. This means that observation is theory-dependent. Einstein supported Popper's view that "theory cannot be fabricated out of the results of observation, but that it can only be invented".[16] Our observations and theories cannot be accepted as objective truth, but must remain open to doubt and reformulation.

A parallel idea is the concept of falsification. Karl Popper teaches that, although one can never succeed in constructing universal truths from a series of observations, at least one can produce hypotheses and seek to falsify, or disprove, them.[17] If I have observed many white swans I cannot conclude that all swans are white, as I have not seen all swans. But a single black swan will falsify the hypothesis that all swans are white. If a hypothesis has survived many attempts to falsify it, I cannot claim that it must be true, but I can claim that it is, at this time, the best available hypothesis. Falsification itself is flawed however. The observational statements that are its key are themselves theory-dependent.

Scientific revolutions

Thomas Kuhn takes a new tack, contending that scientific paradigms do not evolve gracefully as improvements of previous knowledge, but occur as revolutionary events, when enough weight of contradictory observation has discredited a previous paradigm.[18] Kuhn goes further. The weight of evidence needed to endanger an existing paradigm is not determined by scientific logic alone, but also by social and aesthetic influences.

Perhaps the most famous scientific revolution in the 20th century would be the accumulation of evidence that enabled Einstein's theory of relativity to overthrow Newton's hallowed laws. The deep impression left was that if Newton was "wrong" then what now can be regarded as inviolable truth? Fine, Newton may have only been "slightly wrong", but this is reminiscent of the teenager protesting that she is only "slightly pregnant". Newton's laws were perfect and true – and then they weren't.

Relativism

Acknowledging science's inability to lay claim to absolute truth is labelled "relativism". More recently Paul Feyerabend can be seen as an extreme relativist.[19] He claims that, because scientific activity includes subjective methods and the blind chance of circumstance, science has no special claim to represent truth compared with other approaches such as religion or personal opinion.

And what of the content of science itself? At the beginning of the 20th century science could view the universe as composed of predictable little billiard balls, and we knew the rules of the game. All that was left was mopping up. By the end of a century that has seen Relativity, Quantum Mechanics and Chaos Theory (more revolutions for physics than in the previous millennium) science sees the universe as seriously weird and ultimately unpredictable. It's just our 19th-century brains that need to catch up.

Science can no longer make absolute claims to truth. Science can only make claims to a "best buy" model of reality that is stamped with an unclear sell by date. "Reality" is a human construct that will therefore be strongly influenced by the current cultural and historical perspectives. Facts change at an alarming rate these days.

So what of medicine?

Just like science itself, medicine cannot claim a privileged position, with doctors as experts possessed of some refined form of truth. Much of what we do can be shown to have little basis in logic. One example would be that of GPs decision to refer patients to specialists. Moore and Roland pointed out that there is a twenty-fold variation in referral rates between different GPs.[20] A large part of this variation cannot be accounted for by any known variables. Doctors seem to behave unpredictably – surprise surprise! The ultimate subjectivity of medicine is illustrated by two meta-analyses based on the same evidence managing to reach opposite conclusions.[21,22,23] Or again, sometimes our tried and tested methods turn out to be harmful when we actually review the evidence, such as advocating rest for back pain.[24]

Medicine is more closely dependent on technology than on pure science - it is built on what works. And when we compare medical treatment for back pain with "unscientific" alternative practice we do not win.[25] Back pain is a good example of just how poor a science base we sometimes have. Jayson asserts that, with chronic back pain, "in the vast majority of cases it is impossible to identify the source of the pain".[26] And this is for a problem affecting up to 39% of adults.

It is ironic that we pursue biomedicine in the belief it will maximise health. Yet biomedicine has no common agreed method of measuring health status. That is to say, we currently have too many measures, and they are neither coherent nor mutually compatible.[27] Too often we set out, fully trained and armed, in a shiny state-of-the-art jet fighter but with few maps and no way of knowing where the target is.

If our understanding of the world is no longer monolithic but is seen as both relativistic and subject to change, then biomedicine perhaps must become more humble in its claims. It can no longer claim to have a monopoly on the definition of "health". It cannot even claim to be the sole or sovereign source of medical fact. The biomedical model is just that – a model, not an absolute truth. There are other models available. Biomedicine has great strengths, but also limitations. Medicine's methods can be examined for their effectiveness, but medicine must also be more open to public scrutiny of its aims. Experts cannot set these aims in isolation – they are a legitimate subject for public debate and influence.

The limits of biomedicine's success

Case report

Ethel G, a 71-year-old, attended surgery with a sticky red eye for which I prescribed chloramphenicol drops. I noted she had a previous mildly raised blood pressure, and took a further reading, which was about the same. I arranged for the nurse to follow her up according to our practice protocol. She remarked on the way out that what bothered her most was "the screws" – osteoarthritis of her knees, not severe enough to warrant a total knee replacement or stop her from walking, but a daily source of discomfort which she herself manages by simple analgesia and keeping going.

Analysis of consultation outcomes:

1 Prescription for minor, probably self-limiting, condition.
2 Doctor initiated intervention for raised blood pressure, which carries about a one-in-a-hundred chance of benefiting her over a ten-year period, but is not without disbenefit.
3 No effective intervention possible for the one major health problem causing her daily pain and disability.

Perhaps one could see 1980 as the high water mark of medicine's claim to be able to provide universal health. The WHO declared smallpox dead, and served notice of eviction to measles, pertussis, diphtheria and polio. The ink was scarcely dry on the Alma-Ata declaration of the WHO, promising "health for all by the year 2000". And, closer to home, we assumed that the improvement in health of all the UK population would inexorably continue. The explosion of investigation, treatment and cure of the previous few decades would surely continue, enabling us to push back the hold of serious diseases such as ischaemic heart disease, chronic obstructive pulmonary disease, arthritis and cancer.

Then in 1981 we have AIDS. Destined to cause a minor epidemic and much grief in the West, devastation and ruin in parts of the Third World.

One decade later and the WHO's confidence in eliminating further global diseases is looking a bit shaky. In the West a decade of the free market with a shrinking safety net was causing increasing polarisation in health – the rich were getting healthier but the poor were getting iller.

By the turn of the millennium we saw a marked deterioration in the health status of the poorest third of the world. Little news on the WHO hit list. In the West we still have cancer, we still have an epidemic of vascular disease, we still have COPD, rheumatoid arthritis, mental illness, drug abuse, AIDS… The list goes on.

Medicine has succeeded in many of its individual aims. We can do more and more clever things for a minority of peoples' health problems, but the total burden of ill health remains unchecked. The promises of "health for all" from the sixties and seventies lie in ruins.

One of the best known declarations of medicine's impotence comes from the 1970s, from Thomas McKeown, a professor of social medicine at Birmingham:

Literature review

McKeown T, 1976. The Modern Rise of Population. Edward Arnold, London. Chapter 5.

McKeown examines the evidence for crediting medicine with the decline in mortality from the major infectious diseases from the mid-19th century to 1970. He demonstrates that the majority of the decline in mortality occurred before effective medical interventions were developed.

- 86% of the decline in mortality from TB occurred before the introduction of chemotherapy in 1948.
- 93% of the decline in mortality from pertussis occurred before the introduction of immunisation in 1952.
- 82% of the decline in mortality from measles occurred before the most primitive antibiotic treatment of complications became possible in 1935.
- 99% of the decline in mortality from scarlet fever occurred before the introduction of antibiotics.
- The decline in smallpox mortality shows no clear relation to the introduction of vaccination.
- The decline in deaths from cholera, dysentery and typhoid shows no relationship with medical treatment.
- Only for diphtheria is there good evidence that treatment was the cause of the drop in mortality (and even this evidence is not unequivocal).

McKeown's conclusion is that "immunisation and treatment contributed little to the reduction of deaths from infectious diseases before 1935, and over the whole period since cause of death was first registered (in 1838) they were much less important than other influences."

McKeown's thesis provides strong support for the belief that social factors such as housing, income and nutrition have much more effect on health than does medicine.

What does medicine achieve?

We may acknowledge social and environmental factors as the most important determinants of health. We are still left with the question as to how much difference medicine actually makes. One of the most powerful ways of answering the question is the Randomised Control Trial (RCT), surely one of the greatest-ever medical advances in its own right. We search RCTs for statistically significant effects from treatment. But we have a naive tendency to assume that statistical significance implies clinical significance. We have an even worse tendency to assume that a significant effect means we've solved the problem.

Let me illustrate this from a classic trial. In 1985 the MRC reported on their definitive trial of treatment for mild hypertension.[28] Treatment of mild hypertension led to a highly statistically significant effect in reducing strokes ($p<0.01$). This has been widely accepted as evidence that mild hypertension requires treatment. But I would like to use two observations to put the trial in context.

First, although the results are highly statistically significant, their clinical significance remains open to debate. When this trial is quoted the authors' own conclusion is often overlooked: "The trial has shown that if 850 mildly hypertensive patients are given active antihypertensive drugs for one year about one stroke will be prevented. This is an important but an infrequent benefit. Its achievement subjected a substantial percentage of the patients to chronic side effects, mostly but not all minor. Treatment did not appear to save lives or substantially alter the overall risk of coronary heart disease. More than 95% of the control patients remained free of any cardiovascular event during the trial." In other words the deal is that if you take these pills regularly for 30 years there is a less than 4% chance of them preventing a stroke and a 96% chance of it being a waste of time.

So how should we view such treatments? Best we've got? – Yes. Problem solved? – No. Will I benefit if I take it? – Probably not!

But we tend to put a more positive construction on this sort of data. What does this mean? It means spin. Let me list my own perception of likely and unlikely ways of Doctors using this data.

Doctors are likely to say:

- This trial shows that treatment is indicated for mild hypertension.
- Treatment of mild hypertension is effective in preventing strokes.

Doctors are unlikely to say:

- There is a 99.8% probability that treating mild hypertension will do an individual patient no good in any given year.
- Treating mild hypertension fails to prevent the majority of strokes.
- The marginal benefit of treatment must be set against the anxiety, unnecessary medicalisation, side effects and expense of treatment.

And yet all of these statements are valid interpretations of the same results.

We are prone to see the treatment of hypertension as an answer to the risk of CVAs in hypertensives. But treatment fails to prevent the majority of strokes. i.e. it is unlikely to be the solution to the problem. And yet we pose it as the solution because it is the only trick we've got.

Second, the results of the study show that smoking status is a stronger risk factor for CVAs than raised blood pressure. And yet this study is repeatedly cited as support for the treatment of raised blood pressure rather than used as an argument to transfer hypertension clinic money towards broad societal smoking cessation measures.

This suggests we frame our interpretation of trial data in a way that promotes the role of biomedicine as the solution to health problems. We actively select such interpretations of the data even when other conclusions are equally reasonable. To the man with a hammer, every problem is a nail.

The concept of the number needed to treat (NNT) provides another way in. The NNT is the inverse of the absolute benefit of intervention. Chatellier has suggested that NNT is a useful tool for decision-making, as it gives an indication of the likelihood of actual benefit from treatment.[29] But, as Chatellier points out, "what is the clinical meaning of a number needed to treat for five years to avoid one clinical event for the average doctor? Some doctors will probably consider that this number represents an important health benefit, whereas others will consider the benefit as only moderate or even slight".

The SAVE trial shows that if we give captopril after a myocardial infarct then the death rate will fall from 24.7% to 20.4% over three years.[30] This gives a NNT of 23. In other words 23 people have to be treated over three years in order to save one life. This is a genuine benefit that I would not wish to trivialise. However we seldom consider that to obtain this benefit we are treating 22 people without benefit. I would advocate a different measure, the personal probability of benefit (PPB), which is the inverse of the NNT. Thus the PPB for this treatment would be 1 in 23 over three years. One could argue that if we do not explain the low probability of benefit to patients then they are not giving informed consent to treatment.

But where there is clear evidence, how do we use it? Haines and Jones have pointed out that there is often a long delay before doctors implement reliable research findings into their practice.[31] They quote Antman, who found a 13 year delay between meta-analysis demonstrating the value of thrombolytic treatment for myocardial infarction and the incorporation of such advice into review articles or book chapters.[32] The explanation for this is seen in terms of the personal and social processes within the profession. The quality of the evidence base for the treatment a patient receives will therefore depend upon the personality characteristics of the doctor, whether they tend to be an innovator or a laggard. We cannot therefore claim that we consistently use evidence for the benefit of patients. Its use is contaminated by the maintenance of our own medical culture.

Iatrogenic problems

I want to consider this under two headings.

Medical complications

In 1881 US President James Garfield was shot in an assassination attempt. The bullet lodged inside his body. He was a few years too early for an X-ray, therefore a succession of military doctors attempted with unwashed fingers and unsterile probes to locate the bullet. (The evidence for antiseptic technique was by then well established.) The bullet was too deep. The effect of repeated probing was to perforate the liver and cause a suppurating infection. Garfield died 11 weeks later. Post-mortem showed that the bullet was lodged safely in muscle, and that he would have recovered had he been left alone.

If only such horror stories were confined to centuries past. One only has to read the journals of the medical defence societies to see that complications still cause loss and suffering.

How big is the problem?

The honest answer is, we don't know. Iatrogenic problems may be difficult to define, and are often not adequately recorded.[33] This makes analysis difficult, and invalidates many audits. A meta-analysis of prospective studies of adverse drug reactions (ADRs) in US hospital patients showed an overall incidence of 6.7% for serious ADRs, and 0.32% for fatal ADRs.[34] This would make ADRs between the fourth and sixth most common cause of death in US hospitals. A prospective trial in a Chicago hospital gave a rate of 17.7% for all serious adverse events.[35] The likelihood of experiencing a serious adverse event increased by 6% for each day spent in the hospital. A French hospital found that 10.9% of ITU patients had been admitted there due to adverse events, including drug reactions and surgical complications.[36] These patients had a fatality rate of 13%, and cost the hospital $688,470 in medical care in one year. The occurrence of an adverse event more than doubled the risk of death (1.3% increased to 2.9%) in an Australian hospital population.[37]

One consistent message is that ADRs become more likely with increasing age. A study in Tayside showed 5.3% of hospital admissions for the elderly were due to drug ADRs.[38] 66% of these were considered preventable. A US study of nursing home residents found that for every dollar spent on drugs in nursing homes $1.33 in healthcare resources were consumed in the management of ADRs.[39] This was estimated to cost the US $3.6 billion per year. Most iatrogenic disease follows common patterns.[40] It should be prevented, and yet it is not.

We must also remember Davey Smith's cautionary advice.[41] For conditions with a large NNT, only a small minority will benefit from treatment, whereas the disbenefits of treatment potentially apply to each person treated.

When I was younger I made a modest collection of promotional items advertising drugs that had been withdrawn from the market because of safety problems. Zomax, Osmosin, Opren – I had the mugs, the pens, the notepads as memento mori of these once shiny-new but now fallen wonder drugs. Who remembers Practolol, Isoprenaline, Thalidomide, Troglitazone, Tolcapone? Who can tell which items in our current formularies will suffer the same fate?

Diffuse negative effects

This is an area which is harder to quantify than disasters or physical side effects, but it is arguably just as important. Medical intervention can harm peoples' perception of their own health. We treat patients in order to improve their well being, and to reduce disability and suffering. Ultimately these are subjective phenomena. The oldest pillar of medical ethics is to "first do no harm". If I treat a patient's disease but leave them with lower well being and more disability than if I had left them alone, in what way is this a health gain?

This area is examined further in Chapter 7.

What biomedicine leaves out

Case report

Jane is in her 40s. She has terminal multiple sclerosis and insulin dependant diabetes. Virtually quadriplegic she is bedbound and has frontal lobe changes, but she is able to express a clear desire to stay at home. She receives a package of community support, and her aged mother pops in several times a day. Admissions are necessary from time to time, mainly to cope with chest or urinary infections.

After an admission with hyperglycaemia secondary to a UTI she is discharged back home still in a poor condition. She is more drowsy than usual (although her mental state is often difficult to evaluate), and she is not able to swallow fluids. I am called back. As her GP, seeing her carers clearly not coping with her at home, it is easy for me to realise that she was discharged too soon. With the patient's agreement I phone the Medical Registrar responsible for her discharge. He is hostile to the idea of a readmission. I had sent her in with a UTI, hyperglycaemia and early metabolic problems. Her bloods that morning were normal and her urine was clear. Therefore she was fit for discharge.

The purpose of the above case is not to argue for the stupidity or cruelty of Medical Registrars, but rather to show the potential for stupidity and cruelty if the biomedical model is used as a principal source of reality. Iona Heath said in an address to a Regional Educational Conference, "If we only understand the world in biomedical terms we understand very little of it".[42] Biomedicine is a reductionist system, and we can forget that it is the whole person that matters.

There are so many daily examples of our failure to see the whole picture. The patient given a six-week follow-up appointment after a biopsy for a potentially malignant condition. The patient who has waited stoically for nine months for an outpatient appointment only to receive a letter putting the appointment back for a further six months because a clinic is cancelled. The not-so-recent widow whose presenting problem is dealt with but whose grief is left unacknowledged. The patient discharged from casualty late at night in a dressing gown with no way of getting home.[43]

Somatisation

Somatisation means persistant physical symptoms which lead to a belief that one is ill, but in the absence of any physical disease. It is an example of how mind and body cannot be separated into two boxes. It normally represents a bodily expression of repressed psychological distress – physical illness is often seen as more acceptable to the patient and others than psychological symptoms. Somatisation is not malingering. The symptoms are real and troubling enough.

It has been claimed that 20% of GP consultation, with new problems and 30% of referrals to gastroenterology clinics involve somatisation.[44] Grol has shown that treating somatisation within a biomedical model makes patients worse.[45]

The medical gaze

Foucault describes how doctors modify the patient's story, fitting it into a biomedical paradigm, filtering out non-biomedical material.[46] He calls this "the doctor's gaze" – we systematically look at some bits of the story and exclude others.

But surely this is the task of medicine? If I have broken my leg all that matters is what the X-ray looks like and how it can be fixed. If I have bowel obstruction my problems with my boss are irrelevant. This argument fails because most people coming to a doctor do not have straightforward biomedical problems such as broken bones and obstructed bowels. Reality is more complex, and functions on more than one level.

The relevance of the biomedical model to health problems is something like this:

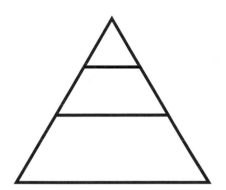

Biomedical model sufficient

Biomedical model insufficient

Biomedical model inappropriate

The reality is of course a continuum rather than nice triangular boxes, but I am trying to give a picture of the bulk of consultations, in which biomedicine is not enough. And even with a clear biomedical diagnosis consider the same problem at three different times:

i   *Biomedical model sufficient:* "Doctor, Johnnie's just fallen off the slide. His leg is bent at a funny angle, and he's screaming in pain."

ii *Biomedical model insufficient:* "Doctor, Johnnie is back at school now on crutches, but finding it difficult. On Monday morning he said his leg was really hurting again."

iii *Biomedical model innapropriate:* "Doctor, Johnnie is out of his plaster now and walking fine, but he's lost his place in the school athletics team. He says he doesn't want to go to school, and last night I heard him crying in his room."

We also see the inadequacy of the biomedical model when we consider the social context of medical problems. Two decades ago the Black Report showed the effect of socioeconomic inequalities on health.[47] One decade later Davey Smith found that social class differences in health were widening, and that the trend was worsening.[48]

The disappearance of the sick man

Literature review

Jewson N, 1976. The disappearance of the sick man from medical cosmology, 1770–1870. Sociology; 10: 225–44.

Jewson describes three phases in the development of Western medical practice:

i   Bedside medicine: this is the traditional relationship between the local doctor or apothecary and the patient, who is seen as a whole person. The problem is defined in terms of the patient's symptoms. A variety of traditional remedies are available, to be purchased at will by the patient as customer.

ii Hospital medicine: the patient is removed from their own environment and put in a hospital bed where the pattern of his daily life is controlled by the doctor. The patient is seen as a case. The prime task of the doctor is the diagnosis and classification of disease. The doctor derives income from his professional career structure.

iii Laboratory medicine: the doctor's focus is to analyse and explain biochemical abnormalities within a scientific model. The patient is seen as a complex of cells with anatomical, biochemical or physiological disturbances. The doctor sees himself as a scientist.

Jewson describes the "disappearance" of the sick man in two senses:

- The patient as a whole person is no longer the focus of medical attention. We have transferred our gaze firstly to organic lesions, secondly to biochemical and physiological disease processes.
- The patient has changed from being an equal participant in a local transaction to being a passive spectator of treatment administered by a powerful and controlling professional class.

The biomedical model has been developed over the last two centuries as a way of fixing what can be fixed. The majority of problems in real life cannot simply be fixed. The biomedical model was developed within hospital medicine. It is more likely to be partly or wholly appropriate for the filtered sample of patients we send to hospital. Even here we cannot assume that a biomedical model is adequate. The triangle may be broader at the top, but the three categories are still there.

In General Practice the majority of cases come into the categories where a biomedical model is either insufficient or even inappropriate. We need therefore to have alternative models to use. It is no use for us to restrict our gaze.

Medical records

Our world is determined (or perhaps created?) by our language. The reliquary of medical language is the patient's notes. I am often aware of the irony of a "good" consultation where I deal with the presenting problem (the baby's snuffles) and then go on to deal with the "real" problem (the strain and anxiety of coping with the demands of a baby with lack of proper support). But I then write in the notes "3/7 snuffles, interferes with feeding & sleep. O/E alert, well++, afebrile, breathing OK, chest nad, E&T nad. Adv & chat & SOS." [GP shorthand for "3 days snuffles, interferes with feeding and sleep. On examination the child is alert and appears generally well, no fever, breathing rate and pattern normal, chest sounds clear, no infection in ears or throat. I have talked about the problem with mum and given her standard advice, but asked her to seek further advice if the child is not getting better normally."]

What are my notes for? If they are to communicate the presenting problem, generate a biomedical construct, and defend me from complaints, then I guess that's fine. If I believe them to be a formulation of how I see the whole problem then I'm kidding myself. Notes tend to distill the pure biomedical model out of the patient's narrative and throw the rest away. Iona Heath said, "If we are to diagnose in psycho-socio-medical terms we need to find ways of recording the data ... Whilst notes are written in biomedical language we are not making a proper diagnosis".[49]

So what is left out? As the state and our own insecurities drive us deeper into the realms of straight biomedicine, humanity gets left out. Care gets left out. Biomedicine is great for fixing biological parts that go wrong. But I am not just the sum of my biological parts. If we believe that people matter then biomedicine is not enough.

Functional aspects of illness

The biomedical model tends to put the mind and the body into separate boxes. True, there is mounting research on the links between the two, but this actually underlines the assumption that they are separate – gee whizz, they are separate but linked!

Disability is a key determinant of health. But disability is a multifactoral construct whose psychological and social determinants are often more important than any biomedical factors.

This area is explored further in Chapters 6 and 7.

The "problematisation of normality"[50]

The WHO defines health as "not merely the absence of disease or infirmity but a state of complete physical, mental and social well-being". But this Utopian vision is an unattainable ideal, bearing no relation to the struggles of real people in an imperfect world. The WHO definition however represents the aim of the biomedical model. We are closed knowable systems, and if something is imperfect it should be fixed. Logically, as none of us is in this complete state of wellbeing, we are all in need of medical intervention to correct whatever "abnormalities" obstruct our path to perfection. But should we view any deviation from perfection as pathology needing treatment? Where do we draw the line?

This problem is explored further in Chapter 7.

Medicine as a target for hijack

Tuckett sees the consultation as a "meeting of experts".[51] The doctor and the patient make an equal contribution. But the interaction between doctor and patient does not take place in a vacuum, but rather within a specific cultural setting. The script could not be transposed unchanged to a different time or place. Society itself acts as a third party in Tuckett's model of doctor–patient decision-making.

The full complexity of our world – its inexhaustible indeterminacy – has been likened by Schon to living in a swamp (see Chapter 2).[52] This feels scary. Society seeks determinacy – it seeks control over the swamp. Evidence-based medicine and surveillance medicine can be looked upon as means of fighting back the borders of indeterminacy, offering control.

A prime tool is the use of guidelines -- maps that make us feel secure that we have found a way through the swamp. They most commonly do this by providing a "best buy" decision algorithm based on data from a biomedical model. This may greatly benefit me if I am suffering a cardiac arrest, but it offers only false illumination if my central dilemma is not biomedical, or is a choice between the utilities of different factors, only some of which are biomedical.

Guidelines also appeal to politicians and Health Service Managers. They hold out the tantalising promise of reducing costs by reducing inefficient management policies and actually preventing future illness. This would be good if it were true. Protocols and guidelines seem to proliferate, however, irrespective of the paucity of evidence that they improve any important outcome measures.[53,54] The sheer quantity of them has led Hibble to describe them as "the new Tower of Babel".[55] Littlejohn found 45 different guidelines for the management of clinical depression, nine from national organizations.[56] The quality of even the national guidelines varied, and this is in a field where a widely respected consensus statement has been made jointly by the Royal College of Psychiatrists and the Royal College of General Practitioners.[57]

Some of the appeal of guidelines is that they may increase the level of control of managers and politicians over both doctors and patients. Before 1990 doctors took their clinical freedom for granted. This is not to say that we have always used it well. None the less it gave us a relatively unfettered setting in which Tuckett's meeting of experts could occur. Each successive round of reforms in the NHS has restricted our freedom to negotiate directly with the patient. Each reform has increased the influence of the ghostly third party in our consulting room.

Maybe this shift in power is inevitable. Medicine cannot be isolated from more general social changes. Other groups are also suffering from state driven deprofessionalisation. Politicians and some sociologists think doctors can't be trusted. So maybe it's even a good thing? But where is the evidence that politicians are more trustworthy than doctors? Opinion polls show that this is not the public's view.

Conclusions

Biomedicine has been a huge success, and has delivered many of its promises. As we make ever greater claims for its universal effectiveness, however, we become aware of its limitations and its side effects. We need to become more realistic about what biomedicine can and cannot achieve. We need to guard against biomedicine becoming a means of social control, whether for the benefit of doctors or of politicians. We need to define what society wants from a healthcare system, and how biomedicine may contribute to this vision.

References

1 The Government's Expenditure Plans – 2000–2001. Departmental Report, Department of Health, April 2000: Chap 3, section 3.2.
2 The Government's Expenditure Plans – 2000–2001. Departmental Report, Department of Health, April 2000: Chap 12, section 12.1.
3 The Government's Expenditure Plans – 2000–2001. Departmental Report, Department of Health, April 2000: Chap 12, section 12.2.
4 The Government's Expenditure Plans – 2000–2001. Departmental Report, Department of Health, April 2000: Chap 12, section 12.3.
5 Pocket World in Figures. London: The Economist/Profile Books Ltd, 1999: p76.
6 Porter R. The greatest benefit to mankind. London: Harper Collins, 1997.
7 Cochrane A. Effectiveness and Efficiency. London: Nuffield, 1972.
8 Hertzler A. The Horse and Buggy Doctor. 1938.
9 Horder, 1949. Quoted in Porter R. The greatest benefit to mankind. London: Harper Collins, 1997: p716.
10 Illich I. Medical Nemesis – The Expropriation of Health. London: Marion Boyars Ltd, 1976. Revised edn: Limits to Medicine. London: Marion Boyars Ltd, 1995.
11 McKeown T. The role of medicine: dream, mirage or nemesis. London: Nuffield Provincial Trust, 1976.
12 McDermott W. Medicine: the public good and one's own. Perspect Biol Med 1978; 21: 167Marion Boyars Ltd,1976–87.
13 Beeson P. Changes in medical therapy during the past half century. Medicine 1980; 59: 79–99.

14 Hadley J. More medical care, better health? Washington, USA: Urban Institute Press, 1982.

15 Chalmers A. What is this thing called Science? Milton Keynes: Open University Press, 2nd Edition, 1982.

16 Einstein's letter to Popper, quoted as appendix to "Logic der Forschung" 1934, translated as The Logic of Scientific Discovery. London: Hutchinson, 1959.

17 Popper K. The Logic of Scientific Discovery. London: Hutchinson, 1959. Popper states "We cannot identify science with truth, for we think that both Newton's and Einstein's theories belong to science, but they cannot both be true, and they may well both be false." Both Popper and Russell acknowledge that Hume (1711-76) "has proved that pure empiricism is not a sufficient basis for science".

18 Kuhn T. The structure of scientific revolutions. University of Chicago, 1962.

19 Feyerabend P. Science in a free society. London: New Left Books, 1978.

20 Moore A, Roland M. How much variation in referral rates among general practitioners is due to chance? BMJ 1989; 298: 500-2.

21 Lindbaek M and Hjortahl P. How do two meta-analyses of similar data reach opposite conclusions? Letter, BMJ 1999; 318: 873-4.

22 Fahey T, Stocks N, Thomas T. Quantitative systematic review of randomised controlled trials comparing antibiotic with placebo for acute cough in adults. BMJ 1998; 316: 906-10.

23 Becker L et al. Antibiotics for acute bronchitis (Cochrane review). In Cochrane Collaboration. Cochrane Library. Issue 1. Oxford: Update Software, 1999.

24 Waddell G, Feder G, Lewis M. Systematic reviews of bed rest and advice to stay active for back pain. British Journal of General Practice 1997; 47: 647-52.

25 Williams N. Managing back pain in general practice - is osteopathy the new paradigm? British Journal of General Practice 1997; 47: 653-5.

26 Jayson M. Why does acute back pain become chronic? BMJ 1997; 314: 1639-40.

27 van Weel C. Of patients and their illnesses. European Journal of General Practice 1998; 4: 3-5.

28 MRC Working Party. MRC trial of treatment of mild hypertension: principal results. BMJ 1985; 291: 97-104.

29 Chatellier G et al. The number needed to treat: a clinically useful nomogram in its proper context. BMJ 1996; 312: 426-9.

30 Pfeffer et al. Effect of captopril on mortality and morbidity in patients with left ventricular dysfunction after myocardial infarction. Results of the Survival and Ventricular Enlargement Trial. N Engl J Med 1992; 327: 669-77.

31 Haines A, Jones R. Implementing findings of research. BMJ 1994; 308: 1488-92.

32 Antman E et al. A comparison of the results of meta-analysis of randomised controlled trials and recommendations of clinical experts. JAMA 1992; 268: 240-8.

33 Geraci J et al. International Classification of Diseases, 9th revision, Clinical modification codes in discharge reports are poor measures of complication occurrence in medical patients. Medical Care 1997; 36 (6): 589-602.

34 Lazarou J et al. Incidence of adverse drug reactions in hospitalized patients: a meta-analysis of prospective studies. JAMA 1998; 279 (15): 1200-5.

35 Andrews L et al. An alternative strategy for studying adverse events in medical care. Lancet 1997; 349 (9048): 309-13.

36 Darchy B et al. Iatrogenic disease as a reason for admission to the intensive care unit: incidence, causes and consequences. Archives of Internal Medicine 1999; 159 (1): 71-8.

37 O'Hara D and Carson N. Reporting of adverse effects in hospitals in Victoria, 1994-1995. Medical Journal of Australia 1997; 166: 460-3.

38 Cunningham G et al. Drug-related problems in elderly patients admitted to Tayside hospitals, methods for prevention and subsequent reassessment. Age & Ageing 1997; 26: 375-82.

39 Bootman J et al. The health care cost of drug-related morbidity and mortality in nursing facilities. Archives of Internal Medicine 1997; 157: 2089-96.

40 Lazarides M et al. Incidence and pattern of iatrogenic arterial injuries. A decade's experience.

Journal of Cardiovascular Surgery 1998; 39: 281–5.

41 Davey Smith G, Egger M. Who benefits from medical interventions? Editorial, BMJ 1994; 308: 72–4.

42 Heath I. Keynote Address. Regional Postgraduate General Practice Educational Conference, South Thames (East). 18th February 1999, Guys Hospital.

43 Anderson C. Saddam strikes in the wrong postal district. Personal view. BMJ 1996; 312: 516–17.

44 Bass C. Article on Somatisation in Medicine on CD Rom. Abingdon, Oxon: The Medicine Publishing Company, 1999.

45 Grol R. To heal or to harm? The prevention of somatic fixation in general practice. London: RCGP Publications, 1981.

46 Foucault M. The birth of the clinic. London: Routledge, 1989: Ch 6. (First published as "Naisssance de la Clinique". France: Presses Universitaires de France, 1963.)

47 Department of Health and Social Security. Inequalities in health: report of a research working group. London: DHSS, 1980.

48 Davey Smith G et al. The Black report on socioeconomic inequalities in health 10 years on. BMJ 1990; 301: 373–7.

49 Heath I. Keynote Address. Regional Postgraduate General Practice Educational Conference, South Thames (East). 18th February 1999, Guys Hospital.

50 Armstrong D. The rise of surveillance medicine. Sociology of Health & Illness 1995; 17, 3, 1995: 393–404.

51 Tuckett D et al. Meetings between experts. London: Tavistock, 1985.

52 Schon D. The reflective practitioner. London: Maurice Temple Smith, 1983.

53 Russell I, Grimshaw J. The effectiveness of referral guidelines: a review of the methods and findings of published evaluations. In Roland M, Coulter A (eds) Hospital referrals. Oxford: Oxford University Press, 1992.

54 Jones R, Lydeard S, Dunleavey J. Problems with implementing guidelines: a randomised controlled trial of consensus management of dyspepsia. Quality in Health Care 1993; 2: 217–21.

55 Hibble et al. Guidelines in general practice: the new Tower of Babel? BMJ 1998; 317: 862–3.

56 Littlejohn P et al. The quantity and quality of clinical practice guidelines for the management of depression in primary care in the UK. British Journal of General Practice 1999; 49: 205–10.

57 Paykel E and Priest R. Recognition and management of depression in general practice: consensus statement. BMJ 1992; 305: 1198–202.

2 Disease versus illness: models in conflict

As the senses never enable us to know things in themselves, but only their appearances, all bodies must be held to be nothing but mere representations in us, and exist nowhere else than merely in our thought.
Immanuel Kant[1]

A proposition is a model of reality as we imagine it.
Ludwig Wittgenstein[2]

We live in a fantasy world, a world of illusion. The great task in life is to find reality.
Iris Murdoch[3]

Chapter summary

We construct a personal knowledge of the world by making mental models. These are closely linked to language itself, and create meaning systems for us. They determine our perception of reality. These models are subjective, and we tailor them to our individual needs.

Doctors use a disease model. This selects different elements of human experience as its building blocks from the patient's illness model. Doctors and patients tend to talk in different languages and therefore live in different worlds. Both models fulfil legitimate but different functions. If we are to be effective in influencing health we need to be able to work fluently within both these models. We need to be open to insights from the social sciences. We need to be aware that there are other models seeking dominance.

The problem of reality

As usual Plato got there first. Two thousand years before Kant he taught that we can have no direct experience of the world itself. We have no God-like comprehension of the billions of particles around us. We do not experience the curvature (or is it now the flatness?) of space, the mutability of time. We cannot know the world. We can only know about the world through our senses.

Furthermore the senses do not report directly to our conscious mind. They are filtered, interpreted and modified by an active process of perception.

Perception is the process through which our mind constructs preliminary internal models out of sensory data. The image on our retina is not the world, it is an image on our retina. One of the few things I remember my anatomy professor saying is "Vision is a punctate system with an illusion of continuity."[4] The beautiful and natural image of the world that is present within our conscious mind is constructed within our brains from a huge body of digital data from the sensory nerves. It is not itself the "real" world. The way the image generated by our brain is present within our consciousness is a miracle and a mystery. This work is not the place to report on the "body–mind problem". To give a childish paraphrase of the argument, does the brain present sensations to the mind – do brain and mind interact? Or is there no separate "mind"? Is our sensation of consciousness an artifact, the result of the colossal complexity of our brain? Books will not answer this question, but will at least show you what a difficult question it is.[5,6,7] The genius of the mind is to create a model of the world which is both useful and, until it is examined more closely, deceives us that it is itself the world.

This separation between the "thing-in-itself" and our perception of it is easily demonstrated by modern neurology.[8] But it is also one of the most important ideas of philosophy. Wittgenstein famously opens his *Tractatus Logico-Philosophicus* with the statement "The world is the totality of facts, not of things".[9] In other words he dismisses the very possibility of talking about the thing-in-itself. We can only talk of "facts", i.e. our own statements of how we find the world to be. St Paul pictures this, and contrasts it with his future hope for the next world: "For now we see through a glass, darkly; but then face to face."[10]

The gap between the world and our perception of it does not end there. We are bombarded with data. We would be overwhelmed if we tried to attend to it all. We therefore have to select aspects of a total sensory experience from which to generate the models that we believe to be relevant to us. We cheat even in this process by relying on cognitive shortcuts, in order to cope with the mass of operational tasks we must perform, and also to cushion the emotional impact of our numerous daily interactions. These shortcuts often have the effect of reinforcing our hypotheses, regardless of evidence, rather than suggesting new ones.

Thinking works by selectivity. I am sitting in my study at a wordprocessor. Most of two walls are taken up by a few hundred books. Most of the other two walls are taken up by 32 pictures, and a window looking over the back garden. My desk is covered by papers, files, journals, computer disks, pots of pens and similar domestic junk. From my window I can see garden. If I sit still, about 10% of my visual field is taken up by my computer screen. If I look around, my screen becomes about 1% of my visual world. And if I gaze into the garden, or open one of the books, then the screen recedes rapidly to the back of my brain. But at the moment the screen and keyboard make up most of my mental world. I say "I'm concentrating". What this means is that, in order to achieve a task, I am ignoring most of the visual stimuli available to me. I am deliberately simplifying my world.

None of us can cope with thinking about the whole world. There are over 10^{11} stars in our galaxy, and about 10^{79} protons in the universe. Any consideration of such totalities is impossible for the mind to grasp, even though, by a strange coincidence, your brain contains 10^{11} neurones. I cannot grasp the reality of the billions of subatomic particles that make up the stapler in front of me. I can only grasp the staggeringly simplified model of it as a "solid" object. I can only cope with this simple object by ignoring most of the facts I know about it and identifying only its task-related characteristic – when I push it, it joins my papers together.

The world we deal with as doctors is complex. What is hidden is, I expect, even more so. We can only deal with the world by ignoring most of it. Then we can select the strands that we need. We can work out how to manipulate such strands into models that represent the world for us. When we get really good at manipulating a defined subset of this totality, we define this bit as "fact".

The swamp of indeterminacy

Schon deals with this issue in his classic book *The Reflective Practitioner*.[11] He uses the metaphor of a swamp to describe the deluge of complex factors that surround any professional problem. In a passage which one could claim as a manifesto for General Practice he states: "In the varied topography of professional practice, there is a high, hard ground where practitioners can make effective use of research-based theory and technique, and there is a swampy lowland where situations are confusing 'messes' incapable of technical solution. The difficulty is that the problems of the high ground, however great their technical interest, are often relatively unimportant to clients or to the larger society, while in the swamp are the problems of greatest human concern. Shall the practitioner stay on the high, hard ground where he can practise rigorously, as he understands rigour, but where he is constrained to deal with problems of relatively little social importance? Or shall he descend to the swamp where he can engage the most important and challenging problems if he is willing to forsake technical rigor?"[12]

So we make sense of our world by making models. A model is a personal map. A map is not the territory it represents, but, if accurate, it has a structure that gives me useful information about the territory. A map represents the aspects of that territory that interest the mapreader. Each of us makes maps that are suited to our own needs. A cabby's map of London will be different from a geologist's map. Neither is wrong. They represent the same world from different perspectives, and they have different uses. These maps are therefore not only personal, but they are designed to be biased – both to our needs and to our comfort.

Epistemology – tough on knowledge, tough on the causes of knowledge

Not only does neuropsychology fit nicely with philosophy at this point, but it also relates to the current philosophy of science as described in Chapter 1. Popper, Kuhn and Feyerabend all, in their different ways, teach that "knowledge" is not a direct apprehension of the world itself. It comes with no guarantee of truth. It is just a current "best buy" model of things. As one author puts it, "truth is stranger than it used to be."[13]

The world is changing fast. Let me illustrate the change through another unlikely historical conversation:

Scene 1. A late-19th-century university common room
Professor of Physics: Well, I think we've just about got the world figured out now. What do you say, old chap?
Professor of Neurology [shuffling awkwardly in his chair]: Er, yes, well, that is to say, we're nearly there. One or two little details to work out, but I'm sure it'll all come out in the wash. We know the truth is out there.
Professor of Philosophy: [Sorry, we are unable to bring you the Professor of Philosophy as the other two won't let him in the same room as them.]

Scene 2. A late-20th-century internet chatroom:
Professors of Physics, Neuropsychology and Philosophy [in unison]: Knowledge is relative to our particular viewpoint, it is provisional and much weirder than we thought.

Language – saying or meaning?

So the story so far goes like this:

world --- ➔ sensory data --- ➔ perception --- ➔ mental model

This will serve us nicely for killing mammoths and hitting tennis balls. As soon as we come to more complex problems such as asking the neighbours round for drinks, or indeed for any issue of meaning, then we need to think big time with our neocortex. To do this we need language. It would be easy to think of language as something that exists to communicate thought. Something that follows on from the thought itself. You try thinking through anything more complex than a simple movement without using language in your mind – it can't be done. Language is more fundamental than communication.

The 20th century has seen an explosion in the study of language.[14] The current story is:

i Language (language as such, not English or French etc.) is an inborn tool for cognitive modelling in the human mind.
ii Language as a communication device is secondary to this, and is partly

an arbitrary system built on top of our innate cognitive modelling language.

iii Only humans have language. (Animals communicate, but they do not have language, only a menu of messages.)

The inbuilt facility for language enables us to be human. It also projects us into a world where we can perceive and create meaning.

Internal language is the tool with which we generate our models of reality. Our models of reality are the only hold we have upon the world. It follows that language is an immensely important determinant of our understanding of the world. Our world and our language are, in a sense, the same thing.

To be meaningful language must be shared. "Supraspinatus" is meaningful to a doctor and "Supralapsarian" is meaningful to a theologian, but not vice versa. Doctors use a medical language that is largely foreign to patients. The implication is not just that we have communication difficulties. We live in different worlds.

Sometimes apparently shared language is deceptive. The human mind creates rich and value-laden associations. Some words are fairly operational and standardised. "This patient has appendicitis" will probably activate a code in your mind something like this: "This patient has an acute inflammatory condition which could lead to a GI perforation and peritonitis. He could die. This is a surgical emergency." Other words are more variable in their significance to the listener. "This child has Scarlet Fever" may imply a benign diagnosis to a doctor, but a sinister threat to a grandmother. Others words may be so emotionally laden as to have completely superseded their operational meaning. Consider the name of a small town in Austria called "Auchwitz".

The changes in meaning that occur between words and the listener's meaning systems are not generally random, but may have recurrent and systematic themes, making these variant meanings into distinct constructs themselves. Roland Barthes calls these constructs "myths".[15] He points out that myths are usually driven by some larger commercial, cultural or ideological motive. To identify the meanings of these myths or symbol systems is to "deconstruct" them – a concept useful in talking about what is going on in a medical consultation.

Back to the real world?

So what has this to do with medicine? Try an analogy. I've talked about the different maps of London that a cabby and a geologist would keep. But what if I'm a generalist? Then I will want an AtoZ, a geology map, a borough and ward boundary map, an Underground map, a tourist guide, and anything else I can lay my hands on. I'm not going to argue that, according to the Ordnance Survey, the Underground plan shows stations in the wrong place. That misses the point. I will value each of them for the parts of the whole picture that together they create. I am also going to update them, because they won't stay accurate for long.

Doctors need to know about biomedical reality. All doctors also need enough people skills to be described as generalists. For GPs generalism is our whole *raison d'être*. If we want to understand people we need to move away from narrow ideologies. We need to know some biomedicine. But we also need to understand people as best we may. We need to understand the mental worlds where our patients live. And to value other academic ways of looking at people and their behaviour.

The time for academic border wars and cattle raids in medicine is over. The 20th century should have taught us that tribalism is a bad idea. Let's get on with the 21st. There are other ways out there of looking at the medical world. If I'm travelling from Catford to Dorset I may need a road map, an AtoZ and also an Underground plan. If I am treating people I need all the help I can get from biomedicine, from the social sciences and from patients themselves.

The rest of this book looks at what we know about how the mental and social worlds of doctors and patients have been constructed. The rest of this chapter looks at a prime area of border warfare: the doctors' world of disease versus the patients' world of illness.

A new model for medical language

I am indebted to my friend Dr Claire Elliott, a North London GP, who drew my attention to a truly inspired paper by Ratzan. By making a bizarre leap of association he gives a fresh viewpoint on the process of being a doctor.

Literature review

Ratzan R, 1992. Winged Words and Chief Complaints: Medical Case Histories and the Parry–Lord Oral-Formulaic Tradition. Literature and Medicine; 11: 94–114.

The big idea of this paper is that medical histories, as presented between professionals, are part of an oral narrative tradition that is distinct from the written tradition, and encompasses different cultures and times. This being the case medical histories can be examined by the same techniques used for other oral narrative works. This paper uses the work of Parry and Lord to compare the narratives of a typical case presentation and Homer's *Iliad*.

The *Iliad* was composed before the invention of the Greek alphabet, and therefore existed exclusively within an oral tradition. In the 1920s Milman Parry, a young Berkeley Classics scholar, developed the Oral-Formulaic theory to explain both the oft-repeated phrases and the inconsistencies within Homer. A formula in this context is "a group of words which is regularly employed under the same metrical conditions to express a given essential idea". The theory envisages that a performer would use a series of formulae (often noun–adjective phrases, e.g. "much enduring divine Odysseus" or "the goddess grey-eyed Athene".) These are then linked together by verbs or brief snatches of free text. As the story would not be written down there would be no chance to re-draft it in a fixed way. (It is not likely that the entire oeuvre would be memorised verbatim.) Rather, within an agreed storyline, the skilled bard would create a recognisable brand of dramatic narrative which would fit semi-automatically within the required dactylic hexameters, all within a live performance that would differ in detail on each occasion. Analysing the first page of the *Iliad* of 168 words, 103 (62%) were within formulae, while 65 words (38%) were free text links.

Parry and his student Albert Lord looked at cultures with a live bardic tradition. They found that the technical demands of such performances produced "a concern with the form of expression, over and above the needs of communication". They found that new bards underwent a semi-formalised system of sitting in, then learning by imitation, and finally singing before a critical audience.

If instead of bardic singing we consider a junior doctor presenting a case on a ward round, and if we substitute senior doctors for tribal elders, then the thesis of this paper is that little of the process would change.

Ratzan points to the ritualistic setting of a traditional "grand round". He points out the stylised form of presentation, with characteristic intonation, gesticulation, pitch, volume and facial control. He notes the similar process of apprenticeship, the similar re-telling of the tale from the patient's first ward round after admission until the history "settles down" on re-telling, re-presentation never identical but approximating to a final form. He points to the increasing distance that develops between this case history and the patient him/herself, whom it is supposed to represent.

What does Ratzan's view mean?

One has little difficulty in demonstrating the formulaic nature of the average case presentation:

> *Patient to doctor:* "Doctor, I've been feeling so tired all the time, and I'm getting these terrible headaches and tingling feelings in my arms. I really don't know why I'm so run down. I'm right off my food. I've been wondering if it's to do with this new microwave my Fred bought me...?"

The "case history" is then edited and remodeled by the student or SHO to conform to an oral formulaic tradition. The underlining indicates the formulaic phrases, which now comprise 30 out of the 42 words:

> *Doctor on ward round one week later:* "<u>This is the first admission of this</u> 47-year-old housewife, <u>with the main complaint of</u> lethargy. <u>She was in good health until</u> three weeks <u>prior to admission, when she experienced</u> lassitude and tiredness <u>of gradual onset. There are associated</u> headaches, anorexia..."

The issue then is: "Whose story is this story?" Ratzan quotes Kleinman: "[Diagnosis] is a thoroughly semiotic activity: an analysis of one symbol system followed by its translation into another. The transmogrification of what used to be a personal story into a set of quasi-scientific, semiquantifiable "facts", signs and symptoms that we call diagnoses ... is a skill we all learn as part of the tradition of becoming physicians."[16] Kleinman describes the metamorphosis of the patient's personal story thus: "Disease is what the practitioner creates in the recasting of illness in terms of theories of disorder ... In recasting illness as disease, something essential to the experience of chronic illness is lost."

There is of course a legitimate need for this reframing for the purpose of some aspects of medical management. Ratzan comments: "The difference between ... interview and medical notation is the difference between illness as the patient's problem and disease as the physician's problem." All trades use their own technical language.

Ratzan also quotes Mishler: "The medical interview may be viewed as an arena of struggle between the natural attitude with its common sense lifeworld and the scientific attitude with its objectified world of abstract logic and rationality".[17] Thus the process of the oral formulaic tradition becomes part of the substance of the final medical history.

Diagnosis as a semiotic activity?

Casting diagnosis as semiotic activity means the translation of the patient's language and meaning system into the doctor's language and meaning system. We tend to picture making a diagnosis as coming to a true understanding of a patient's problem. Rather, we should see it as selecting out the biomedical bits of the problem and rearranging them in a way that enables us to plan a medical intervention. It is not in any sense a "true" understanding of the patient's problem; it is a definition of the bit of the problem that fits our system.

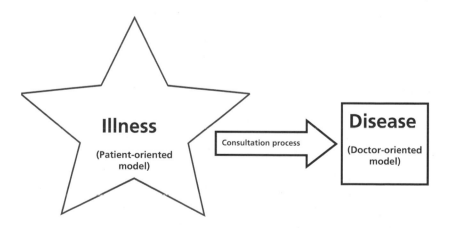

It is rather like scanning a Turner masterpiece into a bitmap picture, and saying that now this is the "true" picture because it is unencumbered by heavy canvas and all that wretched paint. Now I can identify every pixel and send it to you on the internet – it must be better. Yes, something is gained by scanning a Turner into a bitmap, but much more is lost. Let's not kid ourselves that we are dealing with the real thing.

One hopes that the modern consultation bears little resemblance to a grand round. The question remains whether we still blindly remodel the patient's illness narrative or whether we recognise the importance of the illness narrative and seek to recognise it as well as our own disease model.

We do not set out to erase students' understanding of renal function when they move from a medical to a surgical firm. Why then does our system of medical education erase so much of students' lay understanding of illness when they are taught the disease models of the medical tribe? If in medical training one set of language is destroyed then the cognitive world associated with it will disappear also. It is possible to consult in a patient-centred way, but it takes practice.[18]

Disease versus illness

An 81-year-old man made me stop and think. He keeps going, despite his previous splenectomy, recent gastric ulcer and quiescent carcinoma of the prostate. He says: "I don't like going to the doctor. You keep telling me I'm ill."

We know that the models used by doctors and patients may differ. If they did not we would not see so many books on doctor–patient communication. We talk of "the patient's world" and "the doctor's world" as if they are externally determined, given, to be passively encountered by their protagonists. This is not true. Whether we are dealing with a person's experience of illness or a professional's experience of providing health care, our mental model of the world is actively constructed by us from an immense sea of data and a number of possible world models.

It is like being let into a DIY superstore and being told to make oneself a room. I may choose to make a kitchen or an office. Mock Tudor or Star Trek. I may use brick or timber. I have an immense range of choice, and must limit myself to a tiny fraction of the types and quantity of materials available. What I end up with will reflect not so much the materials themselves, but my own personality, preferences and perceived needs.

I must make active choices as I construct my world as a doctor. My choices will rely heavily on the "biomedical" plumbing department of my DIY-World Superstore. Hopefully I will find space for soft furnishings from the humanities department.

The provisional nature of our knowledge is sometimes brought home to us by problematic constructs that won't stay in one piece. Past examples would include "night starvation" and autointoxication due to constipation.[19] There are plenty of current battlefields. Elaine Showalter has collected some of them (including chronic fatigue syndrome, Gulf War syndrome, recovered memory and multiple personality syndrome) together in her wonderful book "Hystories".[20] Summerfield, using the example of post-traumatic stress disorder, points out that we can construct distress and suffering as psychopathology or as normality, according to our own inclinations and culturally related ideologies.[21]

Narrative medicine

One way into the patient's world is through "narrative medicine". This has been described in Greenhalgh and Hurwitz's superb book, *Narrative Based Medicine*:

Book review

Trisha Greenhalgh and Brian Hurwitz, eds. Narrative based medicine. London: BMJ Books, 1998.

This book sees narrative as the bridge between storyteller and listener. It acknowledges the active role of both. As doctors we "construct for ourselves a story about what we think we are hearing".

Narrative is not about general truths, but about the experience of individual people. Narrative contains not only events but also interpretation and feelings.

Patients express their illness experiences within different "narrative streams" than those used by doctors. Patients and doctors therefore assign different meanings to the same events.

Patients' narratives are worth studying because they express the patients' own experience and encourage empathy between doctor and patient, and enable the Doctor to understand the meaning of illness for the patient. Narratives encourage a holistic approach, and may themselves be therapeutic. They encourage reflection. They encourage a patient-oriented agenda and challenge received wisdom.

The medium is the message – the book contains illness stories from writers such as Stephen Jay Gould. There are marvellous chapters on the use of narrative in different specialties, written by the usual suspects such as Iona Heath, John Launer, Marshall Marinker and James Owen Drife.

Narrative is seen as a tool for practising patient-centred medicine. The book tells an important story about what it means to listen to patients. It is one of the most humane medical textbooks you will find. If you have any imagination and any care for patients I would encourage you to read it.

Narrative is a richer concept than the tradition General Practice mantra of "ideas, concerns and expectations" (ICE). ICE is an excellent prompt for us to teach GP Registrars, but the two are not equivalent. It can be sterile if we tack ICE onto an otherwise biomedical model:

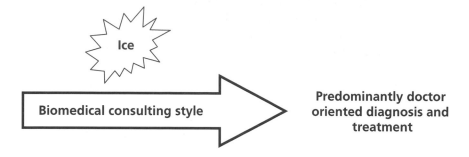

Greenhalgh and Hurwitz encourage us to use the patient's narrative as a legitimate source to contribute to our final understanding of the problem, and as a contributing factor to our management plan. This is not to reject the evident but incomplete benefits from biomedicine.

We could therefore picture the consultation process as having two tracks. The patient initiates a shared narrative element. The doctor constructs and shares a biomedical element:

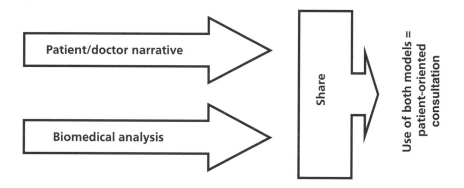

Locus of reality

Lay illness models have roots and connections with the broader range of personal and socially related ideas that make up each individual's world. If we deal impeccably with the doctor's biomedical agenda but fail to address the patient's illness agenda we have failed. Mr A came to see me after his Ophthalmology appointment complaining that the doctor had "done nothing". The specialist had explained to the patient that he had macula degeneration, but had not listened to Mr A's fears and concerns for the future, nor discussed with him why he had the condition.

The justification for the medical model is that we use it to benefit patients. But who defines what benefits patients? If we know our model differs from the patient's then surely we know that only the patient can define what is of benefit, albeit with advice on the technical bits from us.

The issue is one of the "locus of reality" (LOR). How do we define the reality that we will use as a measure of success? Is it the patient's reality or ours? I would suggest that we should pursue outcomes that patients recognise as benefiting them. These benefits therefore have to exist in the patient's world of life experience, not just in our world of biomedical measurements. Especially not just in our world of intermediate biomedical outcomes.

Our models of health and illness are suited to our skills and needs as we function within our world as healthcare professionals. Our patients' models are suited to their skills and needs as members of their own cultural and family groups. Both sets of models give their owners the means to understand what is happening within their own framework of ideas. Both models enable them to know what they should do about most problems that arise. Both are therefore appropriate in their own setting. The patient generally comes to see the doctor when his own explanatory framework is failing to enable him to manage his problem successfully.

General Practice is the jam in the sandwich of lay coping mechanisms and biomedicine. Lay coping mechanisms actually deal with the majority of health-related issues. (What shall I eat today? Shall I try to stop smoking this year? How should I deal with Jason's bruise, my headaches, heavy periods, anxiety about work…?) A minority are brought to the GP, and a minority of these are referred to the hospital medical system:

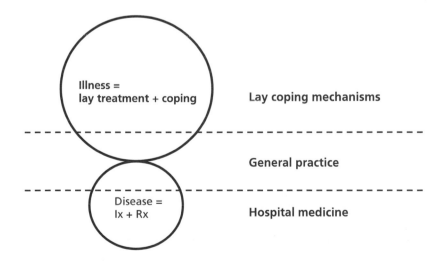

A virtual roleplay

Think through what could happen in the following two consultations. Or grab a friend and try a roleplay for real:

Roleplay 1

You are John Sweet, a 35-year-old insulin-dependant diabetic, diagnosed 10 years ago. You are married with two children. You have got pretty fed up with the fuss doctors make about your diabetes. You get along fine with occasional blood sugar monitoring which tends to be between 10-14mmol/l. You reluctantly agree to attend for annual review, but are worried that the doctor might have a go at you about smoking again. (Your diabetic father smoked 60 cigarettes a day until he died at the age of 67 in an RTA.) You have been told that your blood sugars should be lower. That seems pretty daft to you, because you feel well and none of the bad things that you were told happen to diabetics has happened to you. When you tried to bring your sugars down at the doctor's insistence five years ago you had a couple of hypos which could easily have caused an accident at the garage where you work as a mechanic. The roleplay starts after the doctor has examined you and reviewed your results...

You are Dr Finlay, a new partner in the Wellville Medical Practice. You are seeing Mr Sweet for the first time for a diabetic review. He is a 35-year-old mechanic, an IDDM for 10 years, poor control, last HbA1=10.6%, cholesterol 6.5mmol/l. Microalbiminuria was present at last year's annual review, normal creatinine and BP of 154/90. He smokes 30 a day. Body mass index 31.5. You see from the notes that Mr Sweet is a poor complier with your predecessor's advice. The roleplay starts after you have examined Mr Sweet and reviewed his results...

Roleplay 2

You are Debbie Jones, a 28-year-old lone parent with two lively pre-school children with poor sleep patterns. You live in a one-bedroom flat. You have been feeling very tired recently, and have been having headaches and episodes where you feel weak and get tingling and burning feelings in your hands and feet. Your mum, who lives in Othertown, has told you that it's because you've got weak blood, and she reckons you need a tonic to build you up. She should know, as she has had many different tests over the years for every illness in the book, and she says that the doctors can never seem to find out what's wrong. You have always been slim even though you eat well, and your friend Julie says you look malnourished. Still, Dr Cameron has taken those blood tests, so now you will be able to get something done to sort you out...

You are Dr Cameron, a partner in the Wellville Medical Practice, and have known Debbie Jones since you started her on the pill as a teenager. She is now a harassed lone parent with two pre-school kids. She attended with tiredness, headaches and multiple vague symptoms that you feel are likely to be due to somatisation of her underlying social stresses. You have taken a broad range of screening bloods, which are normal. You see Debbie to give her the results…

In both these situations I have tried to show that the patient's own way of seeing the world is rational, even if not "medically correct". It builds upon their health beliefs. It interrelates these beliefs in a way that makes sense. And that's the point – the patient's model exists to make sense of their world in exactly the same way that medical models make sense in our world.

According to John Fry lay models enable people to cope effectively with 79% of health problems.[22] If you wish to rubbish lay models, do you also want to deal with a five-fold increase in workload? Would people be healthier if they came to you every time they experienced any bodily symptom? Morrell and Whale actually found that, in a group of women aged 20–44, only 3% of symptoms were taken to the doctor.[23]

Most of the time people get on fine without us. They do this by using the explanatory frameworks they already have. These are culturally related and derived from many different sources. Traditional sources include family, upbringing, education and social networks.[24] There is recent evidence that television plays a significant role in forming lay medical beliefs, but with no greater medical authenticity than the more traditional sources.[25,26]

Literature review

Blaxter M, 1983. The causes of disease: women talking. Social Science and Medicine; 17, 2: 59–69.

This is a classic qualitative study, interviewing 46 middle-aged women within a static working-class area. The interviews explored the women's beliefs about the causes of the common illnesses that had affected their families. The categories of causes that were most often cited were infection, heredity, family susceptibility and environmental factors. Degenerative processes were cited less often, as was random chance, which was seen as a frightening concept.

The women's models of disease processes (though often factually incorrect by medical models) contained the same elements as medical models of cause, and were no less sophisticated in their scope.

A causal explanation of illness was clearly important to these women. There was a "strain towards rational explanation and linking together life events". These are "common human traits, which have implications for the interaction between doctors and patients".

The need for parley

In a qualitative paper on patients' experiences of sending for their doctor out of hours, Hopton comments: "The pursuit of a model of out of hours care based on medical necessity that neglects the psychosocial context of illness may not be appropriate."[27] In an editorial comment on the paper Roberts observes that "patients usually have a rationale for actions that may seem to the medical practitioner haphazard, perverse, or plain cussed".[28]

It is banal to fail to realise the role of lay models both in treatment and in coping with the bulk of people's health problems. Even where people need additional help from biomedicine it is futile to believe that we can overwrite patients' own health models and belief systems. (It would be largely destructive if we could.) Rather, there needs to be an accommodation between the lay world and the doctors' world. We need to recognise the value and richness of the lay health world. It provides the explanatory and meaning framework for our patients, and will therefore be the reference point for their coping mechanisms.

When patients come to us ill or in distress we do not make them consult in a foreign language, and then patronise them with praise for their faltering attempts to communicate. Similarly, whilst we need our medical language and world to do the biomedical bits of our job, we should be content for the context of the consultation itself to remain firmly in the patients' world.

I am arguing for Tuckett's "meeting of experts", but I am arguing also that we should develop a greater understanding of the scope and content of the patient's expertise.[29]

Whose model?

If you speak to me in German I will hear only the sounds you make; I will not hear what you *say*. If we do not understand our patients' language and their world then we cannot effectively listen to them. As we have seen, to make a diagnosis in physical, psychological and social terms we must have a language for all three areas. I can only define a problem in terms of my own understanding of the world. If observations are theory-dependent, then diagnoses are model-dependent.

Other models

I have described the importance of lay illness models in the West. I am grateful to my friend Dr Judy Chen for reminding me that the world is not so narrow. In a discussion paper for a local GP research group she mentioned four lay explanatory systems, which see illness as caused by different forces.

Chinese: Illness is seen as an internal imbalance of Yin and Yang forces.
African: Illness is seen as an attack from evil spirits or because of a failure to placate one's ancestors.
Western, historic: Some illnesses are caused by demonic possession.
Western, modern: Based on concepts such as attribution and candidacy (see Chapter 5).

A third way?

The locus of reality for the patient is their own life experience. What happens here defines whether they are ill and whether medical intervention helps. If they feel better then the medicine is OK.

The locus of reality for the doctor in the Western biomedical tradition has been in disease entities. Illness is defined in terms of pathology. Treatment is successful if there is a definable improvement in disease measures. If the disease is treated then the medicine is OK.

There is an increasingly powerful third model competing for dominance. This is the managerial model. It differs from the models of both doctor and patient. Its locus of reality lies neither in illness nor in disease, but in documentation.

I believe this is important. It is more than a trendy doctor finding paperwork a soft target for scorn. It relates to what is my role and what can be used as evidence.

Let me sketch how this model works for General Practice. Before the 1990 NHS reforms General Practice funding came from Family Practitioner Committees. They were headed by an Administrator. In other words the role of the FPC boss was to administer a given contractual arrangement, ensuring that GPs were paid for the work they did within that contract. The GPs were seen as professionals who were, within reasonable limits, autonomous.

After 1990 the FPCs were replaced with Family Health Service Authorities (FHSAs). These were headed by Managers. The role of the FHSA boss now was not to administrate but to manage – to shape the services provided by doctors. The doctor's role is partly de-professionalised. He is not entrusted with the same degree of freedom to practise autonomously, but must provide services as agreed with the FHSA.

The FHSAs were gradually merged into unitary Health Authorities (HAs). These are headed by Chief Executives, with several layers of managers below them. This enables the HAs to implement a far greater level of control over General Practice. There are banding systems, target payment and patronage for local projects for General Practices that are favoured by the HA, and the threat of decreased funding for practices who are not favoured. The doctor is seen as a stakeholder, not as an autonomous professional.

To change a decision made within a model one must have evidence. A patient wants to feel better. A doctor wants scientific evidence about change in a disease process. A manager wants a business plan. Yes, both doctors and managers want patients to feel better too, but there is a difference in the core locus of reality for these three groups as to how we can know whether all is well with the patient.

Since the 1990 reforms, appropriate documentation is the key to obtaining HA support for projects within General Practice. Ideas plus track record cannot compete against good reports and a persuasive business plan.

Over the last decade I, along with many other doctors, have learned to play this new game. It is as if one has to travel to a foreign country and deal in a strange language. One then exports the gains from the deal back into one's own version of the "real world".

There are then three models of the medical world. Each has its own locus of reality, in disease, in illness, and in documentation respectively.

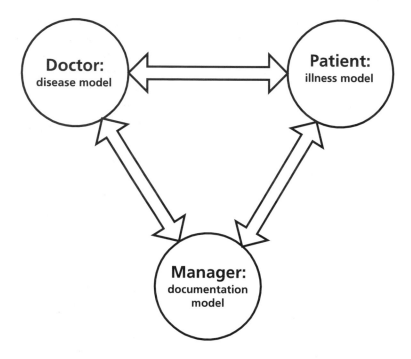

I am not saying that the documentation model is "bad". It is simply a model of reality whose locus is paper. I have no arguments with my own eminently sane HA. I have worked with intelligent, able and humane colleagues to make the pint fill the quart pot. If they were able to come and talk to our 5,800 patients I'm sure they would. But that is the point. They can only deal with a world spun from paper, while I live in a world built of patients and the problems they choose to bring me. If the place of professional decision-making is to be at HA level (population 500,000) then paper must serve as a proxy for patients; there can be no other solution. It may well be that this model is a political inevitability as society invests professionals with less trust and more accountability.

Where is the evidence that a management model of medicine works? James Willis, in his marvellous book *The Paradox of Progress*, argues that increasing systematisation degrades the qualities within a system that are of greatest value.[30]

Willis's thesis is supported by the research we have on patients' priorities:

Literature review

Haigh Smith C and Armstrong D, 1989. Comparison of criteria derived by government and patients for evaluating general practitioner services. BMJ, 299: 494–6.

This study was carried out to evaluate whether there was a consensus between patients' criteria for good General Practice care and the criteria developed by the Government in the white paper "Promoting better health", prior to the 1990 NHS reforms. Twenty-four patients generated 10 quality criteria. These were then mixed with 10 White Paper criteria. All 20 criteria were then ranked for importance by 711 patients.

Rank order	Criterion	Criterion originated by
1	Doctor listens	Patients
2	Doctor sorts out problems	Patients
3	Usually same doctor	Patients
4	Appointment within 2 days	Patients
5	Regular screening for cancer	Government
6	Health checks for adults	Government
7	Staff friendly	Patients
8	Tests done at surgery	Patients
9	Staff know me	Patients
10	Doctor goes on courses	Government
11	Waiting time <20 mins	Patients
12	Small practice	Patients
13	Nurse on premises	Patients
14	Woman doctor available	Government
15	Health checks for children	Government
16	Convenient surgery times	Government
17	Every child immunised	Government
18	Health education	Government
19	Change doctor easily	Government
20	Well decorated premises	Government

Thus only three of the Government's quality criteria were in the patients' top 10. There is evidently a major difference of opinion between patients and the Government as to what constitutes good General Practice.

The lists do not of course compare like with like. Among the top concerns for patients were qualities that are difficult to measure, such as listening. The Government's list consisted of measurable criteria. But perhaps this is the point. As Willis stated, it is the unmeasurable qualities of medical care that are most important. But if Doctors are to be pushed to concentrate on the Government's criteria, doesn't this reduce our ability to deliver the patients' agenda?

The patient priorities found by this paper have been repeatedly supported elsewhere in the literature.[31,32,33] Interestingly Jung found that there is great similarity between the priorities of patients and GPs.[34] This supports the view of Ruta et al, who concluded that properly conducted practice-based needs assessment had great potential for service planning and priority setting.[35]

Priorities mean that some things must take precedence over others. Is it really sane for a publicly-funded health system to give such low priority to those qualities of care identified as most important by the public?

The managerial model tends to take its measures from biomedicine. It will neglect the dynamic of the doctor–patient relationship to reduce a population disease parameter by a part of a decimal point. Even worse, it will do the same to see a marginal improvement in an intermediate outcome, such as the proportion of a population screened.

There are now three models striving for dominance in the NHS. The patient's illness model, the doctor's disease model and the manager's documentation model. They each have their value and place. There is evidence that at least doctors have some connection with the patient's model. There is evidence that the Government (who determine the measures accepted as evidence in the managers' model) have less connection with the patient's model. Is it appropriate that the Government is more firmly in the driving seat of health planning than ever before?

Back to the future

The final irony, of course, comes with Primary Care Groups (PCGs). These once again put doctors in the driving seat, as GPs have a statutory right to be in a majority on PCG Boards. But what professional model are they to use as Board members? They are responsible for developing services in line with Government policy, and within Treasury budgets. They are charged with implementing Clinical Governance, which will exert greater political control over the medical profession than ever before. And will the prime mechanism for decision-making be a reflective chat, considering patients' views and sharing examples of best practice? My friends who are on PCGs tell me it's not like that. A local colleague receives a monthly wodge of A4 paper several inches thick to read in preparation for PCG Board meetings. The doctors may be in the driving seat, but the navigation is to be strictly by management rules. The locus of reality is paper.

It has yet to be seen how things will change when PCGs become Primary Care Trusts (PCTs). Things will move on, no doubt, but take it from me – documentation rules. And that seems set to remain the dominant model of reality.

References

1 Kant I. Prolegomena to any Future metaphysics. Section 13, note II (my paraphrase).

2 Wittgenstein L. Tractatus logico-philosophicus. 1961 translation, Pears D and McGuinness B. London: Routledge. Section 4.01.

3 Murdoch Iris. 'Profile', The Times, 15th April 1983.

4 Warwick R. Undergraduate lecture, Guy's Hospital Medical School, 1974.

5 Popper K and Eccles J. The self and its brain. London: Routledge & Kegan Paul, 1977.

6 Penrose R. The emperor's new mind. Oxford: Oxford University Press, 1990.

7 Pinker S. How the mind works. London: Allen Lane, Penguin Books, 1998.

8 Pinker S. How the mind works. London: Allen Lane, Penguin Books, 1998.

9 Wittgenstein L. Tractatus logico-philosophicus. 1961 translation, Pears D and McGuinness B. London: Routledge. Section 1.1.

10 I Corinthians 13 v 12. Authorised Version.

11 Schon D. The reflective practitioner. Aldershot: Arena, 1995.

12 Schon D. The reflective practitioner. Aldershot: Arena, 1995. p 42.

13 Middleton J and Walsh B. Truth is stranger than it used to be. London: SPCK, 1995.

14 Sebeok T, 1991. A sign is just a sign (Essays). Indiana University Press, USA.

15 Barthes R. Mythologies. Éditions du Seuil, Paris, 1959. Translated 1972 by Annette Lavers, London: Jonathan Cape Ltd.

16 Kleinman A. The illness narratives: suffering, healing, and the human condition.New York: Basic Books, 1988.

17 Mishler E. The discourse of medicine: dialectics of medical interviews. Norwood, NJ: 1984.

18 Stewart et al. Patient-centered medicine, transforming the clinical method. London: Sage, 1995: Chapter 10.

19 Whorton J. Civilisation and the colon: constipation as the "disease of diseases". BMJ 2000; 321: 1586–9.

20 Showalter E. Hystories, hysterical epidemics and modern culture. London: Picador, 1997.

21 Summerfield D. The invention of post-traumatic stress disorder and the social usefulness of a psychiatric category. BMJ 2000; 322: 95–8.

22 Fry J. A new approach to medicine. Lancaster: MTP Press, 1978.

23 Morrell D and Whale C, 1976. Journal of the Royal College of General Practitioners,26: 398.

24 Blaxter M, 1983. Causes of disease: women talking. Social Science and Medicine, 17: 59–69.

25 Gordon P et al. As seen on TV: observational study of cardiopulmonary resuscitation in British television medical dramas. BMJ 1998; 317: 780–3.

26 Walker E. Emergency soaps. BMJ 1999; 318: 744.

27 Hopton J et al. Patients' accounts of calling the doctor out of hours: qualitative study in one general practice. BMJ 1996; 313: 991–4.

28 Roberts H. Listen to the parents. BMJ 1996; 313: 954–5.

29 Tuckett D et al. Meetings between experts. London: Tavistock, 1985.

30 Willis J. The paradox of progress. Oxford: Radcliffe Medical Press, 1995.

31 Wensing M et al, 1998. A systematic review of the literature on patient priorities for general practice care. Part 1: Description of the research domain. Social Science and Medicine, 47: 1573–88.

32 Jung H et al. What makes a good general practitioner: do patients and doctors have different views? British Journal of General Practice, 1997; 47: 805–9.

33 Roberts H and Philp I. Prioritizing performance measures for geriatric medical services: what do the purchasers and providers think? Age & Ageing, 1996; 25: 326–8.

34 Jung H et al. What makes a good general practitioner: do patients and doctors have different views? British Journal of General Practice, 1997; 47: 805–9.

35 Ruta D et al. Determining priorities for change in primary care: the value of practice-based needs assessment. British Journal of General Practice, 1997; 47: 3553–7.

3 How to be a doctor

The first staggering fact about medical education is that, after two and a half years of being taught on the assumption that everyone is the same, the student has to find out for himself that everyone is different, which is really what his experience has taught him since infancy. And the second staggering fact about medical education is that, after being taught for two and half years not to trust any evidence except that based on the measurements of physical science, the student has to find out for himself that all important decisions are in reality made, almost at unconscious level, by that most perfect and complex of computers the human brain.

Sir Robert Platt. British Medical Journal, 1965.

Chapter summary

Doctors are made, not born. We become members of a medical "tribe" with its own cultural norms. Our current system of medical education distances us from the patient's world. Medical language plays a central role in this process. Problems with communication and shared goals are thus inevitable.

Doctors are made, not born

Being a doctor is not an ordinary job

If we invented a doctor's person specification, it might read like this:

- Must be able to break personal and societal taboos by handling and cutting any part of another person's body, sometimes inflicting pain.
- Must be able to carry the daily moral and legal responsibility of making numerous complex decisions, many of which have significant elements of uncertainty, but where any wrong call may cause serious and occasionally fatal outcomes for others.
- Must be empathetic to people with boundless varieties of distress and heartbreak, and be able to help people facing tragedy, loss and death.
- Must be able to do all of the above simultaneously, under pressure, sometimes for very long hours with little support or rest. Must be able to deal with several dozen peoples' needs every day. Must respond equably and without significant slackening of pace when faced with repeated unreasonable expectations and occasional abuse.

Being a doctor is more than a job. We have a distinctive social role. Like being a priest or a lawyer it is a role which often seems to define us. It profoundly influences the way in which others treat us.

To mark this separation, we share with priests the distinction of a title in front of our name – clear product labelling. We form a distinctive peer group. Because we share these powerful experiences, and because the gap between others and ourselves is greater than the gap between most other peer groups, in many ways we resemble a separate "tribe".

By tribe I mean, first, a distinct social group which derives its identity from its own culture, language, social structure and rituals; second, that there is a significant gap between the group and other groups.

Entry into the medical tribe

Becoming a doctor is not just a matter of acquiring knowledge and skills – it is about joining this distinctive tribe. The justification for superseding the patient's "illness" model is that we can use the medical "disease" model to help us to know how to treat the patient best. But Ratzan (see Chapter 2) demonstrates that this operational purpose is not the only reason that the disease model exists.[1] It has also a quite independent root in the cultural rites of the apprentice aspiring to join the medical "tribe".

As I look back on my own initiation into the medical tribe, one turning point for our group was when we became clinical students and first hit the wards in white coats and stethoscopes. A dominant motivation for our learning, as I look back on that time, was our struggle as a marginal group to gain acceptance and recognition as members of the medical tribe.

There were a number of aspects to this. One was the acquisition of knowledge. But this was not so much from a desire to learn how better to help patients. We would have little opportunity to do that for a few years. It was rather to avoid criticism in ward rounds, to get decent grades for each firm, and of course to appease the examiners. A critical part of this process was our performance on ward rounds. We wore the white coat, just as Ratzan's apprentice bard would proudly display his harp. But could we imitate the established tribal members well enough as they effortlessly intoned the mysteries of our craft? Could we move from the margins, to become accepted within the tribe?

Tribes are defined not only by their shared norms but also by their separation from other tribes. I remember the first time I donned a white coat as a very junior student and talked to "a patient". I struggled with how I should behave. I was taken aback by the strange way the patient talked to me, as if I were a member of a different but respected race. There was a guarded intensity, a directedness about our talk that was different from if I had met him in the pub. I struggled to play my part back, not talking naturally but with an earnestness I did not feel, not wanting to let my tribe down. Worse still not wanting him to find out how marginal a member of that tribe I actually was.

In some ways medical students communicate better with patients at entry to medical school than on qualification. They leave the "common sense" world of illness with its complex but partly shared lay illness beliefs that they possess with "patients" and enter the world of the disease models of the medical tribe. Ratzan's paper describes, from an unusual perspective, the process whereby the world that students share with patients is all but erased.

If now I want to become more patient-oriented I face a number of challenges. Ideally I should be able to think within a lay illness model or a medical disease model with equal ease. One model is where the patient lives, the other is where medical treatments are decided. As we have seen in Chapter 2, thinking is inextricably linked to language. I use language to create models of the world. These models are the only way I have of understanding or manipulating the world. If in my training one "set" of language is destroyed then the cognitive world associated with it will disappear also.

Ratzan describes how we learn a new medical language, not for operational reasons but in order to become members of our chosen tribe. If I wish to regain understanding of "the other tribe", that of laity, then reflection on the process of how I became a medical bard will help me to remedy what I lost in achieving that goal. The model looks at the ritual aspects of the struggle between the two worlds, from which the doctor's world emerges.

Of course there is teaching that helps us gain insight into the patient's world. But should we not be seeking a simpler solution? Why does our system of medical education erase so much of a student's lay understanding of "illness" when we teach them "disease"? Surely we should be aiming to teach a model of the patient's problem that encompasses both the patient's illness experience and the doctor's disease paradigm.

We have a legitimate need to belong to the medical tribe by gaining the recognition of our tribal elders. But we have defined ourselves as a tribe in a way that distances us from the patient's tribe. Can we not become more sophisticated in our tribal behaviour to prevent erasure of our lay knowledge?

The medic's progress

We all start our lives in the world of the patient (except perhaps doctors' children). When we go to medical school we leave the lay world, shaking its very dust from our feet, and accept eagerly the overwriting of the medical model. Once practising as doctors we realise our need to communicate across the gulf to our patients, and attempt to reconstruct a lay model as a "second language", as shown on the next page.

Tribal initiation

Dissection has a particular significance in the student's transition from lay person to medic. Dissection is an activity that operates on two levels:

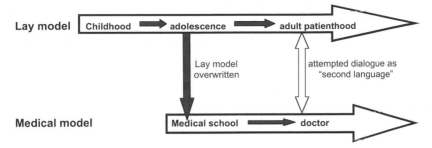

- It is an operational activity, enabling students to learn anatomy.
- It is a ritual, separating the student from the lay world and initiating them into the medical tribe.

Seeing dissection as an initiation ritual is not a new idea. Simon Sinclair devotes a whole chapter of his excellent book *Making Doctors* to the subject.[2] He points out that, along with the selection interview, dissection formed the main subject for question and debate between applicants to medical school and first year medical students at an informal meeting between the two groups. One could see the interview as the rite that qualifies one for admission to the tribe, and dissection as the rite of initiation into the tribe.

Why should we view dissection as an initiation rite? Dissection is an activity heavy with significance. It is a symbol of the student's separation from one tribe and entry into the other:

- Dissection breaks a fundamental taboo of the lay tribe. To cut someone else's body one is either a criminal or a doctor – it is not normative lay tribal behaviour. Both criminals and doctors are excluded from the lay tribe. Dissection is a private activity. TV cameras explore many aspects of education (and every aspect of medicine) but they do not see the dissection rooms. The public is admitted into many parts of the medical school, but not into dissection rooms or the pathology museums. This is *our* territory, *our* secret.
- Dissection presages a fundamental activity of the medical tribe – the handling and therapeutic wounding of other people's bodies. The lay tribe has no difficulty cutting carpets or carving the Christmas turkey, but there is a greater significance in doing the same thing to people. Do you remember the first injection, the first supervised operation during surgical training? Dissection starts our acclimatisation into our new normative world of personal invasion.

Extract from my personal journal, medical school, 1975

I viewed with trepidation the corpse we had been given. He was a wisened old creature, closely resembling an Egyptian mummy. He looked up at us, eyes staring, head back, mouth open as if straining for yet another breath.

He was cold, stiff and like rubber...

Hesitatingly I took up the scalpel and placed it at the beginning of my incision... I paused a second. Perhaps only a few days ago this man had been walking around, laughing wheezily with his friends... There is something within me that cries out "he is human", even though what lies before me is but a puppet without strings...

I inserted the scalpel in a quick shaky motion, and prepared to make my incision. Perhaps he had a wife who is mourning him, remembering with love this thing that lay upon my table... I began to peel the skin back with my scalpel. It is like peeling an orange, except that it requires more mental effort...

The arm ... is duly finished. I get a bone saw to saw it in two at the elbow. This is a Frankeinsteinian job, as the grating edge emerges from the bone to tug jerkily at the remaining flesh, leaving small "crumbs" of skin muscle and bone on the table. The arm duly bisected I put the two pieces in the steel bin.

If you will pardon the juvenile tone, this passage shows what it feels like to be an average 18-year-old from a non-medical home who is told to cut up a corpse. This is a moment of transit.

In the film "Shallow Grave" the task of dismembering a corpse (who had died from an overdose) prior to its clandestine disposal is seen as an understandable cause for one of the characters' subsequent psychological breakdown. Sawing through flesh and bone is portrayed as a psychologically intolerable act. Clearly the circumstances are different – dissection is done by a peer group of volunteers in a ritualistically clinical setting. None the less the act is the same. That this ritual gives entrance to the medical tribe no doubt sustains the student. But still a group of teenagers are expected to spend hours cutting up corpses with no particular recognition that this may be traumatic. One is not supposed to flinch at an initiation ceremony, but there is support to be had from one's peers.

Part of the purpose of an initiation ritual is to prove oneself worthy of entry to the tribe, and to prove that one shares the tribe's mores. After dissection, one is "in".

So what do we know about students' experience of medical school?

Who goes to medical school?

About half of those who apply to medical school will get in. This seems more generous than oft-quoted figures such as "10 applicants per place", but most candidates apply to more than one school. Only students with good A-level prospects will apply. Just under 20% of medical students have a doctor for a parent. Just under 50% of entrants are from social class I, 35% are from social class II, 12% from social class III and 2% from each of social classes IV and V.[2] This has remained fairly stable over a couple of decades.[3,4]

Applicants from ethnic minorities are less likely to be offered a medical school place when compared with white applicants of similar ability.[5] Is medicine "institutionally racist"? Many would say it is.[6,7] The probability of acceptance of such an applicant seems to vary between medical schools in a consistent way year by year. The issue is complex, as ethnic minority applicants (particularly Asian applicants) are actually over-represented in medical schools, compared to those from the general population.[8] The issue in not one of under-representation, therefore, but of equality of opportunity. This is an unresolved controversy that is part of a larger social issue.[9] Medical schools are also less likely to admit applicants who take a gap year, applicants from sixth form colleges, and applicants taking a non-science A-level.[10]

What about idealism?

An unusually high proportion of medical students decide on medicine by mid or late childhood – it seems to be a more fixed career objective than for those pursuing other options.[11] This is associated with medical family members or with an idealistic desire to help others. Many students see medicine as a genuine vocation.[12]

Idealism is a hard quality to categorise. It sounds naive to say at interview "I want to be a doctor because I want to help people." What about the student's immature need to be loved? And yet medicine needs idealists. We should be far more fearful if the research showed we only went into medicine for the money. Youthful idealism needs to become self-aware, mature, more realistic as to what can be achieved. But what disaster if idealism is lost. It is tragic that the idealism of entrants to medical school routinely falters. Johnson and Scott found that 40% of medical students had become cynical about the process and content of medical education by the end of their first year.[13]

Sinclair notes that a persistent linguistic theme among students is the use of irony.[14] Irony is perhaps cynicism criticising itself. It is a traditional coping mechanism for doctors; perhaps a close cousin to the black humour which we use as a defence mechanism, and which seems to stand in for more formal peer support. Irony therefore can be seen as a healthy way of coping internally if it helps us to avoid actual cynicism, and if it is not projected onto our contacts with patients. But these are two big "ifs".

Idealism in the young is a powerful and positive force. But it is seldom free from one's own personal need. When I was a GP Trainee my GP Trainer Dr Manny Tuckman advised me to work out whether I was a doctor who needed to be loved or a doctor who needed to be respected. I protested that I was above such needs – pure altruism all the way. It took me a while, but I discovered he was right. Our struggles in not giving antibiotics for viruses, or in not visiting children with simple fevers, relate mainly to us wanting to feel good. But there is a limit as to how grown up one can be when starting out.

How do students learn?

There can be few other science-based courses where whole blocks of core content such as anatomy have changed little over the last century. Perhaps as surprising is the slow speed of change in teaching methods. Lectures are still seen as the main way for students to acquire a knowledge base. One of the difficulties is the large numbers of students. Twenty years ago the typical medical school intake would be 50–100 students. With the merger of many of the medical schools entry of 200–300 students per year is not unusual. Lectures are cheap and easy to arrange, whilst more modern teaching methods are expensive and logistically more difficult. Could the failure to reform undergraduate medical education be responsible for medicine's failure to modernise its behaviour and attitudes?[15]

One of the big debates is between subject-based learning and problem-based learning (PBL). Do I learn anatomy, physiology, biochemistry, pharmacology, and communication skills, and then magically expect them to integrate seamlessly? Or do I take the new student to a real patient with heart failure and use that as a starting point to which all the individual "ologys" can make their individual contribution?

PBL has become a fashionable answer to the problem of Stone Age medical school methods. PLB has been shown to increase students' enthusiasm for learning.[16] Students find the system less authoritarian (does this mean less teacher-centred?) Students go to medical school to become doctors, not academic scientists. They value early involvement with patients, and early exposure to practical skills.[17]

A central principle of adult education theory is that the learners should take responsibility for their own learning.[18] Medical students find involvement in educational planning improves their learning.[19,20] Doctors have to take more than an average share of responsibility in society, and one might expect that this would be reflected in the methods used in their training. And yet medical education tends to be teacher-, not learner-, centred. Is this then reproduced by doctors becoming doctor-centred instead of patient-centred?

Doctors have to sort out large numbers of facts daily, making decisions that can affect peoples' health, often with large elements of uncertainty woven into the very fabric of the case. Critical thinking skills are essential. Scott found that critical thinking skills only "improved modestly" over the first three years of medical school.[21] Students' Critical Thinking Assessment rating was not correlated with performance during clinical clerkships. Does this imply that much of clinical learning has little to do with thinking?

High pressure learning

The teacher-centred nature of medical education doesn't happen in a vacuum. Particular pressures drive it, which are inherent within the medical curriculum.

The first is the sheer volume of material to be learned. Medical students are traditionally seen to "work hard and play hard". The size of the knowledge base that has to be learned is phenomenal. This problem is then inflated by special pleading from each individual discipline. A committee of Neurologists looking at medical training discovers that students need more neurology teaching.[22] A survey of Rheumatologists concludes that more resources are needed for rheumatology teaching.[23] A review in *Genitourinary Medicine* finds that GUM "merits a greater importance than it appears to receive in current undergraduate courses".[24]

This problem was recognised by the Goodenough report on medical education in 1944. Whilst services for patients have been revolutionised since then, it would appear that services for medical students have not.[25]

The second factor is the issue of responsibility. If I am a bad art teacher the worst that can happen is my students produce something really daft (a bisected cow perhaps?). However, if I fail as a medical teacher, lives are at stake. It's a bit like bringing up teenagers. You know you have to let go, but there is always that sickening worry that they might make a big mistake. The natural tendency, albeit a dysfunctional one, is to dominate, to hold on tight to what is taught. The balance between learning and safety is not easy, as every parent (and every GP Trainer) knows.

Communication skills

There is a famous argument that medical school actually diminishes the student's communication skills. Both Helfer, and later Helfer and Ealy, found evidence to support this view.[26,27] Pfeiffer et al also found evidence that whilst some individual parameters improved there was an overall decline in communication skills over the clinical years in one US medical school.[28] The greatest increase in skill related to interview closure. Such skills are legitimate tools for efficient time management, but can also be used as a way of curtailing the patient's voice. The greatest decrease in skill was in obtaining a social history. Doesn't this sound like students becoming more doctor-centred?

And yet students' consultation skills can be improved with appropriate training.[29] Klamen and Williams showed that ratings remained lowest for students getting patients to ask questions, and answering patients' questions.[30] Again this suggests that students became more skilled in conducting doctor-centred consultations. A survey of communication skills training showed great variation in provision between different UK medical schools, with a lack of infrastructure and support.[31]

It would be hard now to defend the argument that there is a global worsening in communication skills as students progress through medical school. However the evidence suggests that medical school makes students more doctor-oriented in their consultation style. Given that "clerking" is the prime model of the consultation at this stage, this is not surprising. In clerking, one is presented with a pyjama-clad patient on a trolley or bed. The game is to spot the pathology. It is a disease-oriented system that puts little value on the patient's experience and ideas of illness.

Breadth of learning

Garages only matter because they can fix cars. Medicine only matters because it can help people. People are more complicated than cars, but there's a principle in common. What the customer means by "fix" matters. What the customer thinks matters more in medicine, not less, because people are more complicated. Because the only expert on what it is to be myself is me.

It would seem like a good idea for medical students to understand people – as far as possible in an individual, idiosyncratic way. And as much as possible in a more generalisable way. This is the point of the humanities and the social sciences.

Social science is now a standard subject at medical school. Unfortunately there is still evidence that it is there by sufferance. Benbasset found that social science teaching encounters resistance from students.[32] He identified two reasons:

- Students were unsure of the relevance of social sciences for their work as doctors.
- Students perceived negative attitudes to the social sciences from their other teachers.

Thus the ethos of both students and many teachers fails to value the broader "person" part of medicine. This attitude persists beyond undergraduate education – Pabst and Rothkotter found that doctors at the end of their residency saw social science as having little relevance.[33]

I identify peoples' individual idiosyncratic attributes as being important also. This is what McCormick means when he says of James Willis: "He satisfies one of the few important criteria of being a general practitioner, he likes the human race and likes its silly face."[34] But if we have the powerful tools of biomedicine why do we need to bother with individual variability? Why, other than that biomedicine only matters at all if it is of any use to real people. Biomedicine must be chopped down or stretched out to fit people, not the other way round.

So how can we learn about people as individuals? I expect the only satisfactory answer is through life. Through being with other people and finding out what they care about, how they work. Hence the irony of discrimination against applicants who take a gap year – surely the very people who will be more able to relate medicine to the needs of real people.

It seems we don't all have time for life. An academic solution to this problem is the study of literature. Some medical schools in the USA have run classes in literature for medical students for many years.[35] The good news is the British are starting to join in – or at least the enlightened Scots.[36] The claim is that literature can humanise the practice of medicine, by leading to a broader approach than the purely scientific.[37,38] This is seen to aid communication skills, history taking, empathy, ethics and reflection on the doctor's role.

Teaching in general practice

If problem-based learning was the fashionable panacea of the late 1980s then perhaps teaching undergraduate medicine in general practice took on the baton of high fashion in the 1990s.

It is important to distinguish between teaching general practice in a general practice setting and teaching medicine as such. Traditionally medical students spend the bulk of their time in medical schools and teaching hospitals. They have a number of peripheral attachments bolted on, one of which will be in general practice. This is viewed with varying degrees of seriousness by students, but has not been seen as a core part of the course in the same way as being part of a medical firm. As students come out to general practice more often and earlier on in their learning, it would be easy to see this as an increase in GP attachment. It is more significant than this. Brief attachments in the past were to learn about general practice, on the assumption that this is a peripheral branch of medicine. The core of medical learning was seen as the legitimate possession of the medical schools.

Bedside medicine gets even?

Undergraduate teaching in general practice is now going beyond this. The core of medical teaching is no longer the sole possession of the medical schools. As Fry has pointed out, the vast majority of illness happens in the community, and most treatment happens there also.[39] For the focus of medical teaching to move towards the community rather than the teaching hospital is therefore a logical development, but it is more than that. It is the potential reversal of the "disappearance of the sick man" (see Chapter 1). It could prepare the way for the return of a bedside medicine previously displaced by hospital medicine. It gives us a great opportunity to teach a new medicine. Why choose between biomedicine and humanity if we can have both?

Of course I'm getting slightly carried away. This Kuhnian paradigm shift has not happened. But it could.

When I was a medical student in the 1970s medical school was the only possible place to learn medicine. The impression I gained was that most general practice was a poor second cousin to hospital medicine. Sure, a few good doctors went off to be GPs to carry on the family tradition in the leafy shires. But in the city? Nothing good can happen here. Might as well close down the local GPs and deal with problems properly in a teaching hospital – they all come to Casualty anyway.

The first chink of light for me was a miracle worker called Raymond Pietroni. He was rumoured to be doing the impossible – a good general practice that was not in Worcestershire. You could walk down London's Borough High Street from Guy's Hospital and there was a doctor, in a city but not in a hospital, practising intelligent medicine. Of course this was the exception that proved the rule. Except that exceptions were popping up all over the place.

Medical teaching in general practice was seen as impossible when I was a student for various reasons:

- GPs were second-rate doctors.
- GPs didn't have "good cases" – *they* went to the hospitals.
- GPs couldn't teach.
- GPs didn't have the facilities to teach.
- GPs didn't have time – they were too busy giving out sick notes and antibiotics for colds.

So are these problems real, or could general practice become a natural focus for learning medicine?

The rise in the intellectual and personnel base of general practice over the last few decades needs little elaboration. General practice is a mature and attractive specialty. Far from the old cries of isolation, one of its best features is the comradeship experienced within partnerships, learning groups, trainers' workshops, out of hours co-ops, etc. It has pioneered learner-centred teaching methods for GP Registrars. General practice training is surely one of British medicine's most successful medical exports.

But can GPs teach? GPs do teach. Gray and Fine found that 75% of a sample of 310 GPs within the Lambeth Southwark and Lewisham HA had experience of teaching undergraduates, and that 86% of practices had some teaching experience.[40] They found a high level of interest in developing undergraduate teaching further. We are not talking about future possibilities – the future is moving in fast, and deciding on the wallpaper right now.

So, do GPs teach well? Murray et al designed a randomised crossover trial with an endpoint of an objective structured clinical examination to assess whether students could successfully learn clinical method in general practice.[41] In the first six months there was no significant difference in outcome. In the second six months, however, the students taught in general practice scored significantly better. The most conservative interpretation is that GPs can teach clinical skills. And maybe they were modelling communication skills and patient-centred attitudes also.

So what about the patients? The last two decades have swept away the notion of wards full of "good" patients lying passively as teaching fodder for weeks on end. Demographic trends have led to more ill people than ever before. But they are not lying in hospital beds. GPs are looking after them: we know who they are, and we know where they live.

The last two objections are not so easily dismissed. There are real problems with teaching infrastructure, time and money. The infrastructure is developing patchily but none the less rapidly. Gray and Fine identified these as the real issues that would determine the capacity of general practice as a teaching environment.[42] And workload is a problem. It's not that we are too busy giving out sick notes and antibiotics for URTIs. We are too busy doing the real work of chronic disease management that used to be done in outpatient departments, along with our traditional care for minor illness. Wilson et al found that existing clinical teachers in general practice and their partners were enthusiastic about undergraduate teaching, but the majority were unable to increase their involvement:[43] 87% felt that GPs' time pressures had increased after the imposition of the 1990 contract; 88% felt that remuneration for teaching was inadequate – a key factor in enabling the practice to create time for teaching.

General practice could be on the cusp of a revolution in undergraduate teaching. Like any revolution it requires political will and hard cash to succeed.

How do students cope?

Guthrie et al found that 113 out of 172 medical undergraduates showed signs of psychological distress or burnout during at least one of three assessments during their undergraduate training.[44]

Medical training is traditionally seen as being stressful for two reasons:

- The training is long and complex. The knowledge base is large, the standards are demanding and there is a requirement to acquire responsibility.
- Being a doctor is a demanding job. Medical training includes an element of toughening up for the job, and an element of filtering out those who are not up to the job. This has been used as a justification of "teaching by humiliation" and other forms of abuse of students.

A ten-year survey in Leeds Medical School found that 14% of medical undergraduates left their training before qualification.[45] Thirty per cent of leavers cited personal problems, and 8% cited health problems, of which most were mental health problems. This would support the perception of medical training as stressful. Interestingly those who had an A-level in Physics were significantly more likely to leave than those with an A-level in Biology – is it fanciful to think that those with a more deterministic view of the universe found the uncertainties of medicine harder to cope with?

Kamien found that 13% of 4th-year students were "always" anxious.[46] To what extent are anxiety and stress the result of mistreatment or humiliation of students? In a study of US students Richardson found that 37% of 2nd-year and 75% of 3rd-year students reported that they had been subjected to various forms of mistreatment.[47] Mistreatment was lowest in Family Medicine attachments and highest in Obstetrics and Gynaecology and in Surgery.

Rosenberg and Silver describe "medical student abuse".[48,49] This includes "teaching by humiliation", typically on a ward round, where a senior doctor publicly insults and ridicules students or junior doctors. This is damaging to students' morale and self-confidence, and gives a poor model for their own careers as healers and teachers.

Medical education seems to deal harshly with those who become vulnerable. Stewart et al found a vulnerable subgroup of students who become increasingly anxious and depressed from an early stage at medical school.[50] They tend to feel progressively overwhelmed by the workload, and used avoidance strategies to deal with their distress. Simple interventions could benefit this group, but such interventions tend not to happen. Social and cultural adaptation problems may lead on to academic problems.[51]

So how are medical schools doing?

Medical schools are good at some things. Medical schools:

- Produce a constant supply of doctors with a modest drop-out rate.
- Succeed in helping students acquire a huge knowledge base, some of which is relevant for their practice as doctors.
- Succeed in enabling students to acquire many practical skills that they will need as doctors.

Medical schools appear not to perform so well in other ways:

- It is appropriate that entrants to medical school should be able, with a good academic ability. But given that illness is correlated with lower social class, why is medical school entry so skewed towards upper-class entrants? Clearly people from more advantaged backgrounds are more likely to get good A-level results, but this cannot explain the dismally low entrance rates of 12% from social class III and 4% from classes IV and V combined.
- Medical entrants are often idealistic. It would be desirable for this idealism to be explored, matured and fostered, yet it tends to be degraded and replaced by cynicism and irony.
- Communication skills are central to a doctor's job. These are taught patchily, and there is evidence that students move towards a doctor-centred consultation style.
- A broad understanding of people is vital if students are to become mature and humane doctors. Medical schools are still oriented towards producing biomedical technicians.
- There have been huge developments in adult learning techniques in recent decades. Medical schools seem to be at the tail end of

educational reform. They appear to be held hostage by reverence for an inflated knowledge base, much of which is not needed by practising doctors.

- Teaching undergraduate medicine in general practice is a modest success story. It remains under resourced, with major infrastructure difficulties.
- Students are subject to major stresses, and yet are inadequately supported. Mental health problems among students are common. What Bill Styles called "the mask of relaxed brilliance" is a normative way of concealing problems rather than dealing with them.[52]
- Students may be subjected to teaching by humiliation. This is a form of abuse.

So medical schools are good (but old fashioned) at imparting knowledge, good at imparting practical skills, bad at teaching people skills, and disastrous at modelling appropriate humane and patient-centred attitudes. And could it be that we're not getting the right students in the first place?

We enter medical school with a lay understanding of the world. We leave, not with that understanding supplemented by knowledge of biomedicine, but with our lay world overwritten by biomedicine.

Nisker comments: "From the time the medical school's acceptance letter is opened, students eagerly set off on the yellow brick road in pursuit of the attributes of the good physician: intelligence, compassion and courage. The students already possess these traits, just as the Scarecrow, Tin Man and Lion did before they set out for Oz, but they may dissolve in education systems that still decree that the initiation to medicine involve tonnes of tutored words and consuming call schedules."[53]

The medical tribe

So, after emerging from the experience of medical school, what are we like as a tribe? As a group we have a number of characteristics that affect our ability to help patients. Let's look at these one by one.

Dominant

If the medical cosmos was an army, then doctors would be officers and patients would be privates. The medical tribe is a dominant tribe. We control. We stick people on trolleys, we strand them in waiting rooms, and we put them in bed in silly gowns and talk above their heads. We even interrupt a patient's flow of speech after an average of 18 seconds.[54]

There are legitimate reasons for some of our dominance:

- We have an expertise in situations that benefit from a biomedical approach. "Let me through, I'm an Aromatherapist" somehow doesn't sound quite so welcome at a cardiac arrest.

- We are asked by society to work at a rapid pace. One way of making this possible is to control the consultation. To decide for ourselves how much of the patient's agenda to admit. To give out management plans rather than share them. Am I the only one to have an uneasy feeling that I am unable consistently to give patients the quality of doctoring they deserve? There can be a gap between competence and performance. There's nothing like pressure to drive your consulting room through that gap.

The objections to these arguments, though, are obvious. Do we believe in patient-centred medicine or not? The large majority of our consultations are not so biomedically urgent that we have to take over the reins. And are we really saying it's OK to routinely sacrifice quality to keep the NHS going?

Our dominance disempowers the patient. This fits awkwardly with a belief in patient autonomy. Dominance can be even worse than this. It can be depersonalising – making the patient into an object (see Chapter 4).

Doctor-oriented

This characteristic comes from Foucault's medical gaze. We tend to be doctor-oriented because medical school has taught us more about biomedicine than about patients. We tend to use a biomedical model as our main source of meaning, rather than holding the biomedical model and the lay illness model together as parallel and equally valid sources. Being doctor-oriented has consequences on the usual planes:

- Knowledge: using models that relate to our world of disease, rather than the patient's worlds of illness.
- Skills: failing to communicate – the world is in my head, there is no other.
- Attitudes: the job is done once the pathology is named and shamed.

Is there evidence that we are doctor-oriented? Byrne and Long surveyed communication within GPs' consultations in the 1970s.[55] They found that doctors often failed to discover why the patient had attended. (This is not so extraordinary as it appears. If a patient has IBS but is worried they have cancer, it is the fear of cancer not the minor colicky pain that is the reason for their attendance.) They also found that doctors often failed to help the patients to fully understand the problem. Starfield found that, in 50% of consultations, the patient and doctor do not agree on the nature of the main presenting problem.[56]

What follows is a refreshingly honest account of a doctor-oriented consultation.

Record extract

24/5/**

**** Hospital

re: ***** ****** dob: **/**/**

I saw ****** today. It looks as if he has pachyonychia congenita as well as epidermolysis bullosa. There is nothing to be done for these museum specimen diseases. I am afraid I was so interested in this aspect of his case that I forgot to arrange for his warts to be treated. Would you mind, therefore, sending him up again?

Yours sincerely

****

Being doctor-oriented does not only affect the consultation. It affects our understanding of the patient's needs and role. Britten found that hospital doctors holding a strongly biomedical model of illness were less likely to approve of patient access to records, as they did not see the patient as competent to take an active role in the consultation.[57] Jeffery found that A&E staff classify casualties as "good" or "bad" patients, depending on the legitimacy that the staff give to the patient's claim to the sick role.[58] Where the patient's agenda fails to match our own we may resolve the issue by labelling the patient as deviant.

So, have we moved on? There is plenty of evidence that a patient-centred consultation style is not yet the norm.[59,60] Ironically a patient-centred style is very much in the gift of the doctor, not the patient.[61] A patient-centred style requires a fundamental rethink.[62] To treat it as a bolt-on extra is inadequate.[63]

Professional

Professionalism means two things:

- Doctors will perform to adequate standards irrespective of how they feel about a particular task or a particular patient.
- Doctors mostly live in a separate emotional world from their patients.

Performing as a doctor is a learned role. We learn our role from our seniors and from what our patients expect of us.

Suppose I'm having the morning surgery from hell. I call the next patient, Mr Unwashed, who is an aggressive, convicted paedophile presenting with rectal bleeding, and needing a rectal examination. As a doctor I must give this patient the same care, empathy and humane skill that I gave last week, after my shares windfall, to Mrs Niceoldear who runs the local charity shop and who always brings sweets for my kids. This is humanly impossible. But I am not human – I am a doctor. If I cannot produce this same care naturally then I must act as if I could.

But if doing my job involves learning a method of performance, then "I myself" am distanced from the emotions generated within the job. This has both good and bad aspects.

It is good that I am partly distanced from the patient's emotions because I must first attend to my patient's needs within the consultation, not my own. It is no use if I break down and weep when I must give bad news. Patients react to bad news in many different ways: I need to be calmly monitoring their reaction, ready to intervene or move forward according to their needs. The last thing they need is to be burdened with my distress.

I also need to be partly distanced from my patient's emotions for my own protection. Most patients coming to see their GP have some sort of problem, many of which involve distress. I cannot travel an emotional rollercoaster many times a day, week in week out, without risking burnout. My patients' lives are separate from mine, and I need to keep a certain distance for my own wellbeing. I need to respect my own ego boundaries. As Robert Frost said, "good fences make good neighbours."[64]

But there are also times when I do well to use my emotions within the consultation. The Bible exhorts us to "Rejoice with those who rejoice; mourn with those who mourn".[65] The clasped hand, the shared tear cannot be calculated, only judged as to when will be appropriate. The intrinsic emotional intensity and time pressure of the job militate against our ability to use our emotions constructively in the consultation. But if we cannot do our job with humanity then we cannot do our job at all.

Distance

Doctors construct their own reality. Chapter 2 describes how we do this, using the disease model to replace the patient's illness model. We then have to behave within this disease model. Mostly this is not too difficult for us, and simply generates the everyday communication and "compliance" problems that are the commonplace of medicine. There are times when the maintenance of medical reality is harder:

Literature review

Joan P Emerson. Behaviour in private places: sustaining definitions of reality in gynaecological examinations. In Dreitzel H (ed.). Recent Sociology No. 2. New York: Macmillan, 1970.

A vaginal examination (PV) is an example of what Lief and Fox refer to as the privileged access that a doctor has to a patient's body.[66] (They comment that "the physician is permitted to handle the patient's body in ways otherwise permitted only to special intimates, and in the case of procedures such as rectal and vaginal examinations in ways not even permitted to a sexual partner".) In a PV the doctor inserts his fingers into the woman's vagina. But this area of the body normally has a sexual context. This examination is therefore "precarious" in its status as a non-emotive technical procedure.

To remain safe, therefore, the examination must be "constructed" as a medical procedure, removed from the common connotations of such a contact. The examination will usually be conducted in a "medical space". The doctor's behaviour and speech become stylised, as if the doctor as a person is not really there. Eye contact during the examination is often avoided, as if the patient as a person is not there either. Joking is unlikely, and superfluous or lingering contact avoided.

A PV is an example of the clash between the different worlds we construct. Emerson comments that "the gynaecological examination merely exaggerates the internally contradictory nature of definitions of reality found in most situations".

The construction of a medical reality distances us from the patient. This enables the doctor to inflict pain, such as lancing a boil, setting up a drip, or to ask things that cannot normally be talked about.

But this distance is potentially dehumanising to the patient. "Controlled dehumanisation" may be necessary to perform technical procedures. But it may also become a routine way for the doctor to cope with the remorseless pressure of ordinary consultations. This is one of the key features of burnout.

The notes as a surrogate for the patient

If I chat to a friend in a pub, or if I have a business meeting with a colleague, I will look at them; I will meet their eyes. When new GP Registrars first look at videos of their own consultations they commonly discover that they spend a lot of time not looking at the patient but looking at the notes (or computer screen). We may use the notes, written or computerised, as a less demanding patient surrogate. The notes provide a manageable intermediary between the doctor and the patient.

Notes are ideal patients. They are entirely generated by the doctor – no annoying individual eccentricities. They are biomedically oriented. If I write "patient better" then it is so. And they never wake you up at night.

But in the real world we need to attend to the patient. I cannot write "patient better" after some pathological abnormality has been corrected until I have found out that the patient is better.

Pressured

A doctor's job is stressful, and the workload is unrelenting. But we are told that stress is all in the mind – entirely a subjective phenomenon.[67] It is not the external stressors but our inner interpretation of them that makes us stressed. As Epictetus said in the first century, "Men are disturbed not by things but by the views they take of them".[68] One man goes to pieces over his routine desk job, whilst Margaret Thatcher could run the country and defeat Argentina on four hours sleep a night and love it.

Whilst this is clearly true, some situations are harder for the human psyche to endure than others. To take an extreme example, the author Pat Barker showed in her horrifyingly brilliant "Regeneration" trilogy that no one could regard the trenches of the First World War as an unchallenging environment.[69]

Pressure, then, is about what we make of it, but is also about cultural norms. If I had just returned from the trenches I would find civilian life as a doctor to be low in stress. As most of us make less demanding comparisons, relating to Western society's current norms, we are perhaps more justified in feeling stressed.

So are doctors stressed? In the UK in 1994, Caplan found that 27% of GPs scored as depressed or borderline-depressed on the Hospital Anxiety and Depression Scale (HAD Scale), and 14% had suicidal thoughts.[70] In North America in 1998 Sullivan and Buske found a "serious decline in physician morale".[71] A recent BMA report found that 48% of GPs have suffered psychological distress, 14% have felt suicidal and 23% have used alcohol as a response to anxiety.[72]

Burnout and sickness

Does it matter if doctors are chronically stressed? Freudenberger coined the term "burnout" to describe chronic work-related distress.[73] Burnout is usually seen as having three separate but related components. These are:

- Emotional exhaustion.
- Depersonalisation of others.
- Reduced personal accomplishment.

Emotional exhaustion is not only distressing for the doctor; it blunts his ability to recognise and use emotion (his or the patient's) appropriately in the consultation. Depersonalisation means that the doctor treats people (patients and staff) as if they were objects. This is not the best basis for humane medicine. Low accomplishment means less work, and also the vicious circle of low feelings of achievement. So it matters a lot if doctors get burnt out.

Kirwan and Armstrong found that burnout was commoner in UK GPs than in Maslach's North American sample.[74] Worryingly, they also found that some young GPs showed signs of burnout. They questioned whether burnout might be increasing. Sutherland and Cooper had found a reduction in job satisfaction among GPs after the forced introduction of the 1990 contract.[75] The 1990 contract and subsequent changes in UK GP's terms of service have increased GP's workload whilst also increasing direct political control over what we do, thus reducing our own control over our work. Sutherland and Cooper in a further study found a reduction in job satisfaction between 1987 and 1993.[76] They also found a marked increase in anxiety and depression among male doctors, who are more likely to be working full time. This work trend is reminiscent of USA Health Maintenance Organisations (HMOs). Deckard et al found that a staggering 58% of doctors working in HMOs had abnormally high emotional exhaustion scores.

Chronic stress has also been found to cause physical and psychological health problems in doctors.[77] The decreasing level of individual decision latitude is a cause for concern. Two major studies (among non-doctors) of the effect of level of control over one's working environment both found that low control is associated with increased cardiovascular sickness.[78,79]

When doctors do become ill they don't behave like other patients. They rarely go off sick for minor illness or psychological distress.[80] They may not be registered with a doctor themselves, and often self-medicate with prescription-only medicines, including psychotropic drugs.[81] In a study of UK doctors 87% reported that they had worked when they felt too unwell to carry out their duties to the best of their ability.[82]

Alcohol, drugs and suicide

Medical students and hospital juniors are less likely to abuse drugs than the rest of the population of the same age.[83,84] But then things change. Doctors are more likely than others to die from diseases caused by alcohol.[85] Doctors are also at increased risk of drug addiction. In an Australian study 0.4% of doctors had their authority to administer opiates withdrawn over a ten-year period due to detected drug abuse.[86] The prevalence of substance abuse or dependence over the span of a doctor's career is approximately 10–15%.[87] Drugs are easily available to stressed doctors. A study from the Maudsley Hospital found that only 5% of doctors who misused drugs used the black market for their supplies.[88] A Canadian study found that 8% of hospital doctors were using self-prescribed psychoactive medication.[89]

Suicide rates among doctors are higher than those in the general population, and higher than those in similar academic groups.[90] A systematic review of population-based studies found that male doctors are about twice as likely, and female doctors about four times as likely to commit suicide compared to the general population.[91]

Does it matter to patients?

Schattner found that when GPs were stressed patient care suffered.[92] Firth-Cozens and Greenhalgh found that over a third of hospital doctors and general practitioners reported specific instances where patient care had been compromised through tiredness, overwork and depression.[93] Seven percent of these incidents involved serious errors, and two incidents resulted in avoidable patient deaths. And 25% of UK GPs plan to take early retirement because of the NHS reforms and increased patient demands.[94]

The facts suggest that, as a profession, we are more likely to become ill, burnt out or depressed than our patients, and yet we are likely to respond to these problems by denial, self-treatment, addiction or suicide. The medical culture is not good at caring for sick doctors. This is not good for us, and it's not good for patients.

Conclusion

An ideal healthcare system would have workers readily able to empathise with the ill by having a similar background, and an understanding of the patient's illness world. Medical schools select students from the subgroup of society least associated with illness, and then remove any lay understanding of illness they might have from them.

An ideal healthcare system would be patient-oriented, would value autonomy, be empathetic and give time and space for humanity. Doctors are inducted into, and then perpetuate, a system that is doctor-oriented and under pressure. This squeezes out the patient's needs and the patient's ability to contribute to their system of care.

Doctors care for their patients, and yet we are bad at caring for ourselves despite increased risk of damage. Sick doctors will not make well patients.

References

1 Ratzan R, 1992. Winged words and chief complaints: medical case histories and the Parry–Lord Oral-Formulaic tradition. Literature and Medicine; 11: 94-114.

2 Sinclair S, 1997. Making doctors. Oxford: Berg, Ch 7.

3 McManus I and Richards P, 1984. Audit of admission to medical school: I – Acceptances and rejects. BMJ; 289: 1201-4.

4 McManus et al, 1995. Medical school applicants from ethnic minority groups: identifying if and when they are disadvantaged. BMJ; 310: 496-500.

5 McManus I, 1998. Factors affecting likelihood of applicants being offered a place in medical schools in the UK in 1996 and 1997: retrospective study. BMJ; 317: 1097-8.

6 Esmail A and Everington S, 1993. Racial discrimination against doctors from ethnic minorities. BMJ; 306: 691-2.

7 Esmail A, Everington S and Doyle H, 1998. Racial discrimination in the allocation of distinction

awards? Analysis of list of award holders by type of award, specialty and region. BMJ; 316: 193–5.

8 Esmail A, 1998. Commentary: League tables will help. BMJ; 317.

9 Abbasi K, 1998. Editorial. BMJ; 317: 1149.

10 McManus I, 1998. Factors affecting likelihood of applicants being offered a place in medical schools in the UK in 1996 and 1997: retrospective study. BMJ; 317: 1097–8.

11 Allen I, 1988. Doctors and their careers. London: Policy Studies Institute.

12 Sinclair S, 1997. Making doctors. Oxford: Berg. Chap 4.

13 Johnson A and Scott C, 1998. Relationship between early clinical exposure and first-year students' attitudes towards medical education. Academic Medicine; 73 (4): 430–2.

14 Sinclair S, 1997. Making doctors. Oxford: Berg. Chap 5.

15 Maudsley R, 1999. Content in context: medical education and society's needs. Academic medicine; 74 (2): 143-5.

16 Kaufman D and Mann K, 1996. Comparing students' attitudes in problem-based and conventional curricula. Academic Medicine; 71 (10): 1096-9.

17 Ward B et al, 1997. The views of medical students and junior doctors on pre-graduate clinical teaching. Postgraduate Medical Journal; 73 (865): 723–5.

18 Rogers A, 1988. Teaching Adults. Milton Keynes: Open University Press.

19 Huppatz C, 1996. The essential role of the student in curriculum planning. Medical Education; 30 (1): 9–13.

20 Fafowora O, 1996. Can medical students design their ophthalmology programme? East African Medical Journal; 73 (6): 407–9.

21 Scott J et al, 1998. Critical thinking: change during medical school and relationship to performance in clinical clerkships. Medical Education; 32 (1): 14–18.

22 Charles P et al, 1999. How much neurology should a medical student learn? A position statement of the AAN Undergraduate Education Subcommittee. Academic Medicine; 74 (1): 23–6.

23 Kay L and Walker D, 1998. Improving musculoskeletal clinical skills teaching. A regionwide audit and intervention study. Annals of the Rheumatic Diseases; 57 (11): 656–9.

24 Jones G et al, 1996. Venus and Freud: an educational opportunity? Genitourinary Medicine; 72 (4): 290–4.

25 Ministry of Health and the Department of Health for Scotland, 1944. Report of the interdepartmental committee on medical schools (Goodenough report). London: HMSO.

26 Helfer R, 1970. An objective comparison of the paediatric interviewing skills of freshmen and senior medical students. Pediatrics; 45: 623–7.

27 Helfer R and Ealy K, 1972. Observations of paediatric interviewing skills. American Journal of Diseases in Childhood; 123: 556–60.

28 Pfeiffer C et al, 1998. The rise and fall of students' skill in obtaining a medical history. Medical Education; 32 (3): 283–8.

29 Evans B et al, 1996. Consulting skills training and medical students' interviewing efficiency. Medical Education; 30 (2): 121–8.

30 Klamen D and Williams R, 1997. The effect of medical education on students' patient-satisfaction ratings. Academic Medicine; 72 (1): 57–61.

31 Hargie O et al, 1998. A survey of communication skills training in UK schools of medicine: present practices and prospective proposals. Medical Education; 32 (1): 25–34.

32 Benbassat J, 1996. Teaching the social sciences to undergraduate medical students. Israel Journal of Medical Sciences; 32: 217–21.

33 Pabst R and Rothkotter H, 1997. Retrospective evaluation of undergraduate medical education by doctors at the end of their residency time in hospitals: consequences for the anatomical curriculum. Anatomical Record; 249: 431–4.

34 McCormick J, 1995. Foreword to Willis J. The Paradox of Progress. Oxford: Radcliffe Medical Press.

35 Poirier S, 1991. Towards a reciprocity of systems. Literature and Medicine; 10: 66–79.

36 Calman K et al, 1988. Literature and medicine: a short course for medical students. Medical Education; 22: 265–9.

37 Downie R et al, 1997. Humanizing medicine: a special study module. Medical Education; 31: 276–80.

38 Smith B, 1998. Literature in our medical schools. British Journal of General Practice; 48: 1337–40.

39 Fry J, 1979. Common diseases, their nature incidence and care. Lancaster: MTP Press: Ch 3.

40 Gray J and Fine B, 1997. General practitioner teaching in the community: a study of their teaching experience and interest in undergraduate teaching in the future. British Journal of General Practice; 47: 623–6.

41 Murray E et al, 1998. Can students learn clinical method in general practice? A randomised crossover trial based on objective structured clinical examinations. BMJ; 315: 920–3.

42 Gray J and Fine B, 1997. General practitioner teaching in the community: a study of their teaching experience and interest in undergraduate teaching in the future. British Journal of General Practice; 47: 623–6.

43 Wilson et al, 1996. Undergraduate teaching in the community: can general practice deliver? British Journal of General Practice; 46: 457–60.

44 Guthrie et al, 1998. Psychological stress and burnout in medical students: a five year prospective longitudinal study. Journal of the Royal Society of Medicine; 91: 237–43.

45 Simpson K and Budd K, 1996. Medical student attrition: a ten year survey in one medical school. Medical Education; 30: 172–8.

46 Kamien M and Power R, 1996. Lifestyle and habits of fourth year medical students at the University of Western Australia. Australian Family Physician, Suppl 1: S26–9.

47 Richardson D et al, 1997. Assessing medical students' perceptions of mistreatment in their second and third years. Academic Medicine; 72: 728–30.

48 Rosenburg D and Silver H, 1984. Medical student abuse. An unnecessary and preventable cause of stress. J Am Med Assoc; 251: 739–42.

49 Silver H and Glicken H, 1990. Medical student abuse. Incidence, severity and significance. JAMA; 263: 527–32.

50 Stewart S et al, 1997. Predicting stress in first year medical students: a longitudinal study. Medical Education; 31 (3): 163–8.

51 Schreier A and Abramovitch H, 1996. American medical students in Israel: stress and coping. Medical Education; 30 (6): 445–52.

52 Styles W, 1993. Stress in undergraduate medical education : 'the mask of relaxed brilliance.' British Journal of General Practice; 43: 46–7.

53 Nisker J. The yellow brick road of medical education. Canadian Medical Association Journal 1997; 156(5): 689–91.

54 Frankel R and Beckman H, 1989. Evaluating the patient's primary problem(s). In Stuart M and Roter D (eds), Communicating with medical patients. Newbury Park: Sage: pp. 86–98.

55 Byrne L and Long B, 1976. Doctors talking to patients. London: RCGP Publications.

56 Starfield B et al. The influence of patient–practitioner agreement on outcome of care. American Journal of Public Health 1981; 71: 127–131.

57 Britten N, 1991. Hospital consultants' views of their patients. Sociology of Health and Illness; 13 (1): 83–97.

58 Jeffery R, 1979. Normal rubbish: deviant patients in casualty departments. Sociology of Health and Illness; 1 (1): 90–107.

59 Eggly S et al, 1997. An assessment of residents' competence in the delivery of bad news to patients. Academic Medicine; 72 (5): 397–9.

60 Joos S et al, 1993. Patients' desires and satisfaction in general medical clinics. Public Health Reports; 108: 751–9.

61 Street R et al, 1995. Increasing patient involvement in choosing treatment for early breast

cancer. Cancer; 76: 2275–85.

62 Barnard D, 1985. Unsung questions of medical ethics. Social Science and Medicine; 21 (3): 243–9.

63 Butler C and Rollnick S, 1996. Missing the meaning and provoking resistance; a case of myalgic encephalomyelitis. Family Practice; 13: 106–9.

64 Frost R, 1957. "Mending Wall". From Ten Twentieth-Century Poets. London: Harrap.

65 St Paul's letter to the Romans, Chapter 12 verse 15, New International Version of the Bible. London: Hodder and Stoughton, 1973.

66 Lief H and Fox R, 1963. Training for detached concern in medical students, in Lief H et al (eds). The psychological basis of medical practice. New York: Harper and Row.

67 Ogden J, 1996. Health Psychology: a textbook. Buckingham: Open University Press. Ch 10.

68 Epictetus. As quoted by Blackburn I and Davidson K in Cognitive therapy for depression and anxiety. Oxford: Blackwell Scientific Publications, 1990: Ch 2.

69 Barker P, 1992. Regeneration. London: Penguin.

70 Caplan R, 1994. Stress, anxiety and depression in hospital consultants, general practitioners and senior health service managers. BMJ; 309: 1261–3.

71 Sullivan P and Buske L, 1998. Results from CMA's huge 1998 physician survey point to a dispirited profession. Canadian Medical Association Journal; 159: 525–8.

72 BMA Working Party, 2000. Work related stress among senior doctors. London: BMA.

73 Freudenberger H, 1974. Staff burnout. Journal of Social Issues; 30: 159–65.

74 Kirwan M and Armstrong D, 1995. Investigation of burnout in a sample of British general practitioners. British Journal of General Practice; 45: 259–60

75 Sutherland V and Cooper C, 1992. Job stress, satisfaction and mental health among general practitioners before and after the introduction of the new contract. BMJ; 304: 1545–8.

76 Sutherland V and Cooper C, 1993. Identifying distress among general practitioners: predictors of psychological ill-health and job dissatisfaction. Social Science and Medicine; 37: 575–81.

77 Schattner P, 1998. Stress in general practice. How can GPs cope? Australian Family Physician; 27: 993–0.

78 Marmot M et al, 1997. Contribution of job control and other risk factors to social variations in coronary heart disease incidence (The Whitehall II study). Lancet; 350: 235–9.

79 Johnson J et al, 1996. Long term psychosocial work environment and cardiovascular mortality among Swedish men. American Journal of Public Health; 86: 324–31.

80 Waldron H, 1996. Sickness in the medical profession. Annals of Occupational Hygeine; 40: 391–6.

81 Wines A et al, 1998. Surgeon, don't heal thyself: a study of the health of Australian urologists. Australian and New Zealand Journal of Surgery; 68: 778–81.

82 Waldron H, 1996. Sickness in the medical profession. Annals of Occupational Hygeine; 40: 391–6.

83 Baldwin D et al, 1991. Substance use among senior medical students. A survey of 23 medical schools. JAMA; 265: 2074–8.

84 Hughes P et al, 1992. Resident physician use by speciality. Americal Journal of Psychiatry; 149: 1348–54.

85 Brooke D, 1997. Impairment in the medical and legal professions. Journal of Psychosomatic Research; 43: 27–34.

86 Cadman M and Bell J, 1998. Doctors detected self-administering opioids in New South Wales, 1985-1994: characteristics and outcomes. Medical Journal of Australia; 169: 419–21.

87 Bohigian G et al, 1994. Substance abuse and dependence in physicians: an overview of the effects of alcohol and drug abuse. Missouri Medicine; 91: 233–9.

88 Brooke D et al 1991. Addiction as an occupational hazard: 144 doctors with drug and alcohol problems. British Journal of Addiction; 86: 1011–16.

89 Lutsky I et al 1994. Use of psychoactive substances in three medical specialities: anaesthesia, medicine and surgery. Canadian Journal of Anaesthesia; 41: 561–7.

90 Lindeman S et al 1997. Suicide mortality among medical doctors in Finland: are females more prone to suicide than their male colleagues? Psychological Medicine; 27: 1219–22.

91 Lindeman S et al 1996. A systematic review on gender-specific suicide mortality in medical doctors. British Journal of Psychiatry; 168: 274–9.

92 Schattner P, 1998. Stress in general practice. How can GPs cope? Australian Family Physician; 27: 993–8.

93 Firth-Cozens J and Greenhalgh J, 1997. Doctors' perceptions of the links between stress and lowered clinical care. Social Science and Medicine; 44: 1017–22.

94 BMA Working Party, 2000. Work related stress among senior doctors. London: BMA.

4 How to be a patient

Illness is the night-side of life ... Everyone who is born holds dual citizenship, in the kingdom of the well and in the kingdom of the sick. Although we all prefer to use only the good passport, sooner or later each of us is obliged, at least for a spell, to identify ourselves as citizens of that other place.

Susan Sontag,Illness as Metaphor, 1978.

The ultimate indignity is to be given a bedpan by a stranger who calls you by your first name.

Maggie Kuhn, The Observer, 20 Aug 1978.

Chapter summary

Vulnerability due to illness and subsequent treatment by doctors turns people into patients. Patients are active in coping with their illnesses, but doctors tend to treat the patient as a passive recipient of care rather than engaging with them as an active agent.

Them and us

Let's start with an extract from a BMJ "Personal View", by Felicity Reynolds, a professor of obstetric anaesthesia in London:

Personal view

Felicity Reynolds. Personal view. BMJ; 312: 982–3. (With permission from the BMJ Publishing group.)

Are hospital patients fellow human beings?

"Of course they are," you cry. Yes, we all agree they are human beings, but the question is, are they fellow human beings? ...

On a recent sailing holiday, forgetting my advancing years, I made too hasty an effort to jump off our boat on to the quay. One leg slipped between the railings of the pulpit from which I found myself dangling, having smashed my lateral tibial condyle. Pausing in the local hospital only for x ray examination, backslab and analgesia (supplied with efficiency and kindness) I hot footed it to the familiar surroundings of my own hospital. Of course I had the red carpet treatment and went swiftly between ward, x ray department, operating theatre, recovery room, ward, x ray department, etc.

I then discovered an interesting fact. I have worked at this hospital on and off for 40 years and know literally hundreds of faces. Yet now, wheeled around in a bed, I had become mysteriously invisible to friends and colleagues encountered by chance in corridors and lifts.

Moreover, I found that even my voice had become inaudible. I made one visit to the x ray department in the early postoperative days, feeling ill with a chest infection as well as pain in the knee and iliac crest (donor area). I also had a contracted bladder following continuous catheter drainage. As time passed I began to think myself abandoned as I believe many patients do in x ray departments. Eventually feeling desperate and spotting a friendly consultant radiologist, I called, "Jim". No response and he disappeared around the corner. Later he passed again. "Jim", I called more loudly. Again he carried on. A third time I saw him and shouted, "Jim". A puzzled look came on to his face and he paused and looked round at head height. Again I called, "Jim" and waved frantically hoping his eye would stray down in my direction. Thank heaven it did and he finally saw me. I asked could he very kindly make something happen as I was feeling rotten. "Oh dear," he said, "you are having NHS treatment." This made me feel rather ashamed, but from then on my visit to the x ray department went smoothly and swiftly.

After three weeks of convalescence I returned to work part time on crutches. Everybody was unfailingly helpful, opening heavy swing doors, etc. But to colleagues and friends around the hospital who did not know of my situation, I remained invisible. I tried wearing a white coat – largely ineffective. It was not until four months after the injury, when I was able to hobble about without crutches, that my body gained substance. As I limped around the hospital friends would say, "Good heavens, whatever has happened to you?" At last I was a fellow human being.

I read the BMJ starting from the back. Minerva, books, "Personal Views" and columns, and of course the obituaries. And yes, I do read the papers – the "real" contents, the academic bit. The British Journal of General Practice is even more explicit in its intellectual apartheid. It relegates the swapping of yarns to a special section called "The Back Pages" (its use of capitals.) And yet, I am told, The Back Pages were introduced to make the Journal more readable, and perhaps more read.

So what is the "real" content of a medical journal? What is the "real" content of our medical model? Or what is the "real" content of the patient's complaint? In this book I am seeking to redefine the medical gaze. If we simply pick out the patient's biomedical bits we do them a disservice. A holistic picture of the patient themselves is not just a fashionable and intriguing addition to our work, but surely it is our work. But "personal views" and clinical narratives are arranged in the BMJ in a way that clearly shows them to be subsidiary to the "real" function of the journal.

Felicity Reynolds's "Personal View" is one of many that illustrate the perspective transformation that is experienced when one becomes a patient.[1,2,3,4] Before describing this transformation it is worth stopping to note just how common a theme this is in BMJ Personal Views and elsewhere. (The American College of Physicians runs a similar column in the Annals of Internal Medicine. A collection of these has recently been published in book form, and is well worth reading.[5]) The doctor becomes a patient, and suddenly: "hey – I've made an amazing new discovery – the patient's world is different!"

I cannot enter anyone else's world, but surely I can learn about it? Can I only understand the needs of a patient with a broken leg if I have suffered the same injury myself? The point of Dr Reynolds's story is that in writing it she believes that we might share at least something of what she learned.

So what happens when a person turns into a patient? How can we who, by and large, are not patients, learn about the patient's world? Well, we have the broader literature from other disciplines. And we have a wealth of narrative, both written and from our own patients. Is this information legitimate to our medical minds? Does it lie within the medical gaze? If it doesn't, perhaps it is time that it did.

The academic literature examines the process of becoming a patient from a number of different perspectives.

Who becomes a patient?

As Sontag points out in the quote at the top of the chapter, we are all potential patients. But some are more likely patients than others. One might think that people go to a doctor if they experience any symptom that might indicate illness – a simple stimulus/response model like this:

symptom of possible illness ⇒ see doctor

But this nice Pavlovian model is wrong.

Literature review
_____

Zola I. Pathways to the doctor: from person to patient. Social Science and Medicine 1973; 7: 677–89.

This classic paper demonstrates that becoming a patient is a more complex transition than it appears – it's not just about attending to a disease. Zola asserts that "the very labelling and definition of a bodily state as a symptom, as well as the decision to do something about it, is in itself part of a social process."

Minor physical symptoms are universal daily experiences, and more significant symptoms are common, with only the minority taken to a doctor. Zola contends that patients "accommodate", physically and socially, to symptoms. Patients consult a doctor not when they get a symptom, but when their "accommodation" to the symptom breaks down. This "trigger" leads the patient to seek help.

Zola identifies five types of trigger:

- The occurrence of an interpersonal crisis.
- The perceived interference with social or personal relations.
- Sanctioning – being given "permission" to attend by family or friends.
- The perceived interference with work or physical activity.
- Time limiting of symptomatology – "If it doesn't get better in a week I'll see the doctor".

Much of Zola's paper relates to the different ways that illness will present in different ethnic groups. He studied Irish, Italian and Anglo-Saxon patients presenting with new problems at an outpatient department in Boston, USA. Irish patients were more likely to present with symptoms localised to one anatomical site, and complain of interference with bodily functioning. Italian patients were more likely to present with diffuse symptomatology and pain.

If Zola is right then there is much more to going to see the doctor than being ill. It is an activity more akin to booking a course, full of implications and social connections, than buying more bread because I have run out. This process occurs against a background of changing norms and expectations. In 1971–72 66% of the total population visited their doctor at least once - this increased to 78% in 1991–92.[6] As well as demographic change there is an increasing medicalisation of life.

This social dimension is emphasised by Zola's finding of ethnic differences in presentation. Our perception and evaluation of symptoms are culturally influenced. This can be most clearly seen in the presentation of non-specific symptoms indicating underlying psychosocial dysfunction. In my own practice I have observed that a young or middle-aged white Western patient may complain of being "tired all the time", whereas a patient of Asian origin may complain of a widespread burning sensation, or a patient from Africa may complain of "pains all over".

There is therefore a large non-biomedical element in how symptoms are perceived, and in what symptoms are considered significant enough to bring to the doctor.

Literature review

Mechanic D and Volkart E, 1960. Illness behaviour and medical diagnosis. Journal of Health and Human Behaviour; 1: 86–94.

This classic paper coins the term "illness behaviour". This means "the ways in which given symptoms may be differentially perceived, evaluated, and acted (or not acted) upon by different kinds of persons".

The study measured the tendency of people to adopt the "sick role" when presented with non-specific and probably minor symptoms. The research confirms that people with a high tendency to adopt the sick role were over-represented among those attending a doctor. They found a particular excess of high sick role tendency patients presenting with gastrointestinal complaints and minor injuries.

The study also examined the effects of perceived stress on illness presentation. High perceived stress was positively associated with an increased tendency to adopt the sick role. There was also a positive relationship between high perceived stress and allergies, minor trauma and skin conditions.

The illness presented to doctors is not a representative sample of the total burden of illness in the population. There is an over-representation of minor illness presented to doctors from a subgroup within the population with an increased tendency to adopt the sick role. This subgroup is also more likely to suffer from gastrointestinal complaints and minor injuries.

The authors conclude that people do not attend the doctor simply as a result of discovering disease. The decision to seek medical care depends on a number of factors, only some of which are biomedical. Personality traits and perceived stress are also important. Any analysis of illness as seen by doctors must take into account psychosocial as well as biomedical factors.

Case report

Horace was a retired professional man in his 80s. He was single with no close family, little in the way of medical history, in possession of his faculties but quite frail. He lived in a large house, cared for by an elderly housekeeper. He would frequently request home visits for trivial symptoms. We came to an unspoken understanding that I would visit him on about one telephone call in three, which meant I would visit perhaps a couple of times a month. All suggestions of ways of getting out and socialising, or of improving diet or care arrangements were politely ignored.

One day he developed crushing central chest pain. When he became sweaty and short of breath the housekeeper became concerned, and asked if she should call me (the first time she had ever suggested this action to him). He refused this suggestion, and duly died of his first myocardial infarction a couple of hours later.

Clearly Horace represents an extreme case, but he illustrates the fact that whatever it was that he used to call me for it was not because of a Pavlovian response to the presence of a symptom. There is much more in the process of deciding whether or not to become a patient than the possibility of disease.

If a person decides to see a doctor, and if that doctor feels that more than a brief assessment or minor intervention is required then the person's life changes as they become a patient. Let us consider the characteristics of this transformation.

Brody has a fictional Chief of Medicine declare that "To be sick is to feel dependant and childlike, to feel unwhole, broken, defective. To be sick is to be robbed of basic self-esteem, to feel powerless to do what everyone else can do without hesitation or effort … They say that we doctors reduce our sick patients to dependence and passivity by our arrogance and authoritarianism. But why should we bother when the sickness has already done it for us?"[7]

It is arguable how much of patients' dependency is caused by doctors and how much is inherent, as Brody's Chief claims, in the experience of being ill. I guess it takes two to tango.

Illness can represent a personal crisis. As Moos and Schaefer have said, "An acute health crisis is often a key turning point in an individual's life. The vivid confrontation with a severe physical illness or injury, prolonged treatment and uncertainty, and intense personal strains can have a profound and lasting impact."[8]

When a patient becomes acutely ill, the doctor must respond with an appropriate action plan. In the case of a heart attack a Medical Registrar may order an ECG, Chest X-ray, blood tests, put up a drip to administer pain relief and streptokinase. With an acute illness it is therefore easy to think of the patient's role as passive, but this is not the case. Patients have their own active responses to make to the acute threat of illness. Moos and Schaefer identify seven adaptive tasks that patients need to perform.

1 Dealing with symptoms, such as pain and disability

Acute symptoms can be scary, especially if the patient is alone. Doctors judge seriousness by pathology rather than symptoms, but patients do not have this source of potential reassurance. For a passenger in mid-flight a loud bang followed by a lurch would make most passengers aroused and scared that the plane might crash, even if the pilot knows things are under control. Similarly for patients dizziness or weakness may mean loss of control, imminent collapse or a fit. Palpitations may mean the heart might stop. Shortness of breath may imply death by suffocation or choking.

If I get a symptom, what action should I take? Most symptoms do not imply clear-cut responses, as we shall see further in Chapter 5. Most symptoms involve suffering, and coping with loss, whether just loss of a day's work from flu, loss of a limb from blocked circulation, or impending loss of life from cancer. We tend to remember Elizabeth Kubler Ross's five-stage model of a loss reaction in relation to bereavement, but in fact her model was developed from talking to dying patients themselves.[9] Denial, anger, bargaining, resignation and adjustment may all be present in any loss reaction, small or great.

Disability suddenly looms much taller when it affects oneself. Limbs or sense organs not doing what they should suddenly turn the normal acts of living into an assault course. The energy needed to cope with all these challenges can be great, and this is only the beginning of the story. Sick people are rarely passive, but they may be overwhelmed.

2 Dealing with treatment procedures (and perhaps hospitalisation)

This might mean anything from enduring a needle or an internal examination to learning to cope with a colostomy bag or home dialysis. Here we are citizens of Sontag's "other place".

Hospitalisation, by Sontag's analogy, is like being dumped in a foreign land where we know little of the language, and where the locals dominate us. In terms of our ability to act we are highly dependant, but we are not passive. We are climbing rapidly up a learning curve in order to cope with a changed life and regain some control.

Consider the technical requirement of completing tasks which may increase in their difficulty if one is ill. Attending outpatients in a Regional Centre may not seem a daunting task to a doctor, but getting on and off unfamiliar trains may be hard if you are frail, confused by complex new environments and feeling ill.

3 Developing relationships with healthcare staff

This "other place" is well populated with the medical tribe and its allied families of nurses and paramedical staff. They got there first and arranged the furniture to their taste. They are well intentioned but none the less they are a distinct tribe with their own customs. And they have power over what will happen to you. Your relationships will be mostly friendly but also tinged with anxiety and misunderstanding.

A relationship of trust under these circumstances will always be partial, and will always contain a certain tension. How safe is it to express frustration or anger? How safe is it to express one's own wishes when the experts have their own plans?

And of course the patient will have to get used to dealing with many healthcare staff. "I never see the same doctor twice" is perhaps as common a complaint now in primary care as it used to be in outpatients. There is always an inequality of power. The patient needs the medics, and the relationship proceeds on the medic's terms.

4 Preserving an emotional balance

There are many negative emotions associated with illness. As well as direct suffering there may be a sense of guilt, sometimes appropriate (if only I hadn't taken that bend in the road at 60) or mostly inappropriate (what did I do wrong to have this miscarriage?). There may be a sense of failure (the heart attack means that even if I get back to work I won't do the overtime and so I can't now pay the mortgage). There may be threats to the self of anxiety and alienation.

These sort of negative emotions are not helpful when the patient has to fight the effects of illness. It is all the more important for the patient to deal with these feelings in order to regain some optimism and hope for the future.

5 Preserving a satisfactory self-image and maintaining a sense of competence and mastery

If we are to live our lives effectively we need to maintain a sense of mastery over our world and ourselves. The patient may need to accept help when they are ill, but there is a difficult balance. We need the sense that, within known boundaries, we are able to will and to act as we feel best. If this crumbles, then our ability run our lives competently and autonomously is threatened.

Self-image may be damaged by scarring, disfigurement or disability. This is another sort of loss needing adjustment and acceptance. If patients have lost the ability to earn or to care for others they may feel inadequate. There may be apprehension for the future.

There may need to be changes in personal values and lifestyle. If an early-middle-aged patient's picture of himself is as young and able, then illness may challenge this. Can he find a way to be OK as not so young, and not so able? If part of the self-image is feeling attractive how will he cope on the beach with a surgical scar? Just like the pre-illness life itself, self-mastery has to be re-built.

6 Sustaining relationships with family and friends

Illness brings change within families. Many patients are children, carers or wage earners. Here especially there will need to be major adjustments to how the family works. Even if the patient is none of these things they are still likely to be part of some family network.

Illness therefore presents families with unwelcome change. The family network must adjust. The family may need to cope with loss of income, loss of skill capacity or loss of future prospects and hope.

7 Preparing for an uncertain future

We know we cannot know the future, but we tend to live as if we can. We have to structure our lives. If the SWOT (strengths, weaknesses, opportunities, threats) analysis of our lives suddenly changes then we have to reconstruct our hopes and fears.

Most illnesses carry a degree of uncertainty. "When will my rheumatoid arthritis come under control?" "How long will my postviral fatigue last?" "Will I be well enough to take my exam on Friday?" "How long have I got, Doc?" The only truthful medical answer to such questions is "I don't know".

Uncertain hope is frustrating, even tormenting. As John Cleese said in the film "Clockwise", "It's not the despair – I can cope with the despair. It's the hope I can't stand."

An ill patient may be many things, but they are not passive recipients of medical care. They are pedalling hard to keep up. They are actively adapting to illness and reconstructing their world. These may be difficult tasks that may interfere with their physical recovery if they do not go well. Doctors therefore need to be aware of the patient's work, in order to facilitate it if this is needed.

This is not to say that all patients need counselling. It *is* to say that all patients need humanity, consideration and kindness. A few will need more than this, and if the doctor or other medical staff cannot provide the necessary help then counselling may well be appropriate.

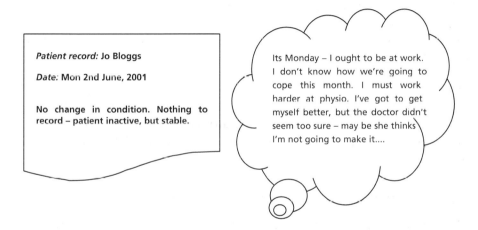

Patient utilities

This rather inelegant expression means "what matters to the patient". Well of course that's easy, surely they want to get better? But as medics we know it's not as simple as that.

Every option, every outcome will have different meanings and different values for different patients. Extreme examples are obvious. To me the risks involved in a blood transfusion are acceptable if they will save my life, but not to a Jehovah's Witness, whose religious beliefs forbid transfusion. To me the minor perils involved in vaccination are well worth it for the gain of protecting my children from the killers of a century ago. But not to a specialised subgroup of anxious parents.

These examples depend upon the very differing belief systems that we have within a free and pluralistic society. More important however are the differences in values and priorities that we all possess. Consider the following list of problems that could happen to you over the next year:

- Myocardial infarction
- Infertility
- Epilepsy
- Total deafness
- Panic disorder
- Osteoarthritis of the knee
- Loss of an eye
- Need to take long-term medication
- Bereavement
- Depression
- Below knee amputation of a leg.

If you ask any group of apparently similar people to score how bad each event would be for them on a scale of 1 to 10, you will get a surprising degree of divergence.

To a professional footballer a knee injury may be the worst thing that could possibly happen. To a politician or manager a heart attack may prevent further career progression. If personal appearance is a key part of self image (or earning capacity) then a glass eye may score worst. To a person with high and rigid expectations of self (perhaps a doctor) a mental health problem may seem like the end of the world. I have seen patients scarcely affected by bereavement, and others devastated, never to recover.

We all have our own priorities, and we all have different ways of constructing an acceptable image of ourselves. We all have different relationships and things we value. Illness may pose threats to:

- Self image
- Relationships
- Social function
- Comfort
- Earning ability
- Future goals
- Expected lifespan.

To assume that we know the significance of a diagnosis to an individual patient is just as daft as assuming we can guess the diagnosis as they walk through the door. We make a diagnosis mainly by talking to the patient. We can try to understand the patient's world by the same method, but we have to work at it.

Can we use patient utilities?

Medical decisions rely not just on scientific evidence but also upon human judgements about the relative importances of different outcomes. These judgements are subjective. For example, to one patient protection from osteoporosis by ten years of HRT may be worth the 6 per 1000 increase in the risk of breast cancer, but for another patient any increase in cancer risk may make the treatment unacceptable.

Patient utilities apply not only to major long-term treatments, but to the decision whether to take any treatment we advise. Patients are not passive. They evaluate the doctor's actions. They appraise the value of the treatment from their perspective, and balance this against the perceived negative effects of medication. There may be a number of concerns, such as:

- Fears about taking "a drug".
- The expense of prescription charges.
- The inconvenience of remembering medication, especially at work or school.
- The negative effects of accepting an illness label.
- The fear of stigma from illness.
- Side effects of medication.

It is difficult to measure and record patient utilities, but that doesn't mean they don't matter. Some attempts to do so have been made.

Von Neuman devised the "Standard Gamble".[10] This balances the negative utility of a particular outcome against a risk of sudden death. It demonstrates what risk a patient is prepared to take in order to achieve (or avoid) a particular outcome. Torrance devised the "Time Trade-off".[11] This defines the value of improvements in health status by comparing them to the amount of life expectancy an individual is prepared to forgo to achieve them.

It is difficult to know whether these are valid ways of comparing high probability/low disbenefit states with low probability/high disbenefit states, which is the choice facing a patient contemplating routine treatment to modify risk factors.

Literature review

The impact of patients' preferences on the treatment of atrial fibrillation: observational study of patient-based decision analysis. Protheroe J et al, 2000. British Medical Journal; 320: 1380–4.

Would patients make the same treatment decisions about anticoagulation for atrial fibrillation as doctors if they had access to the same risk–benefit evidence? This is a multicentre GP study based on interviews with patients aged between 70 and 85 years suffering from AF.

Anticoagulation with warfarin gives a 68% relative risk reduction in strokes due to AF. However not everyone with AF would get a stroke, warfarin does not prevent all strokes, and warfarin itself may have side effects, sometimes serious. When the probability of each of these different outcomes was explained to patients only 61% elected to be anticoagulated, although the guidelines suggest that over 90% of this group should be anticoagulated.

82 of the 97 patients expressed a preference to be involved in shared decision-making. The large majority found it quite acceptable to discuss stroke risk, although 22 found it "a little" unsettling, and 2 found it "very" unsettling. A weakness of the study is that of 195 eligible patients only 97 completed the decision analysis process.

This study shows three things. First, it is practical to involve patients in complex decision-making (but not necessarily within a ten minute consultation!) Second, not all will choose to take part. Third, it makes a difference when we do involve patients.

Smeeth, in a commentary on Prothero et al's paper, comments "Good clinical practice can ... be informed by the evidence; it may not always follow the evidence".[12] Beauchamp and Childress point out that "beneficence provides the primary goal and rationale of medicine and health care..."[13] Beneficence means doing good. But "good" in this context is highly subjective. One man's good is another man's poison. There are often choices between different good or not-so-good outcomes. Only the patient can determine what is the best buy for them. Proper medical goals should therefore normally be seen as patient-defined and subjective. Outcomes that patients want are more important than outcomes that doctors can measure.

The fly in the ointment of patient choice

As any pollster or politician knows, a major difficulty in getting patients' views is the effects of "framing" on the questions asked. "Would you take a treatment that will reduce your risk of a stroke by 45%?" may be the same question as "would you take a drug that had a 97% probability of doing no you good?", and yet it is likely to produce a different answer. This is because it is drawing on different parts of a medical model of risk, and by choosing a particular perspective one can profoundly influence the answers.

Patient narratives

In Chapter 2 I argued that we should attempt to listen to the patient's own accounts of their experience of illness. We need to listen to their experience of receiving healthcare services also.

Letter from a patient

I have been in hospital more than a dozen times and I am deeply grateful for the care and attention I have received. However I have noticed that over the years there has been a decline in hands-on nursing... I had trouble last time in to get the one night nurse to help a crippled lady in the next bed crying with cramp. The nurse simply told her off for not lying in the right position and I had to get up and go and seek her out again before she would give the crippled lady anything to ease the pain. However most nurses do care. I well remember a male nurse who showed wonderful care for an elderly patient who was dying.

Administration is very muddled. When I first saw the surgeon he wanted me to have three tests and then come to see him again. I duly got [three dates] the last of which was well after the date I was to see the surgeon! After seeing the surgeon again I finally got a letter telling me, in the first paragraph, to report to the hospital ward at 9am. The second paragraph said I was first to ring up the ward between 9 and 9.30am to see if there was a bed available for me!

On the ward at one time there was a lady opposite me who was having oxygen. The machine failed, an alarm went off and I remember the sight of six nurses gathered round the machine not knowing what to do, not one of them looking at the old lady and all too intent to hear another patient calling for a bed pan.

I cannot help feeling that we should sack all the remote managers and bring back the matron. We need to plan around "small is beautiful", less university degrees and more hands-on caring, less management from afar and more on-the-spot leadership. Despite all the kindness and treatment I received I feel the NHS has deteriorated over the years.

I have chopped four paragraphs from this letter, but it is otherwise exactly as written. How do we deal with this sort of narrative? Certainly one could answer the individual criticisms, referring to staff business, minor glitches that could be corrected etc. One could comment that the patient was not justified in drawing such a sweeping conclusion from her individual experience. But this would be to fail to recognise the chasm in culture and gaze that is explicit in this patient's story. This is an account of a reality that we cannot deny – the reality of one patient's experience.

We can learn about the world on the other side of this gulf by listening to patients' narratives. By listening, I mean more than hearing the words. I mean seeking to comprehend the model of the world that is conveyed. And I mean recognising the legitimacy of that model too.

If you want some patient narratives to practise listening to, let me recommend three:

Book review

Diamond J, 1998. "C". London: Vermilion.

John Diamond is a journalist. This is his account of the problems of diagnosis of his carcinoma of the tongue and of the almost unbearable treatments that followed. It is honest, funny, excruciating and endlessly enlightening. It is very readable. Diamond manages to convey something of what it is like to be a patient, in the middle of a life, struggling with illness.

It is a meaningful account of an "ordinary" serious illness, such as many of our patients face daily. After 20 years as a doctor few books have taught me more about what it is like to be a patient.

Book review

Bauby J, 1997. The diving bell and the butterfly. London: Fourth Estate.

Bauby was the French editor of *Elle*. In 1995 he suffered a massive CVA, leaving him with "locked-in syndrome" – fully retaining his mental faculties but speechless and totally paralysed apart from the ability to move one eyelid.

This is an exceptional book. Within 139 pages of brief chapters, each dictated by blinking his eye, Bauby reflects on his past, on his present, and on the effects of his condition on his family. Bauby creates a unique testimony of the limits of the human experience, perhaps comparable only to works such as Primo Levi's *If this is a man*. The analogy of the title refers to the frustration of the butterfly of his mind trapped within a heavy unresponsive dead diving bell of a body.

Few patients experience anything approaching the horror of Bauby's illness, but he reminds us of the mystery and absurdity of what it is to be human in a malfunctioning body.

Book review

McCrum R, 2000. My year off. London: Picador.

Robert McCrum is literary editor of *The Observer*. He suffered a severe stroke at the age of 42. He comments: "I was treated incredibly well throughout". But he also says, "Whenever I speak to fellow stroke sufferers, it is this frustration, bitterness, rage – call it what you will – that surfaces most quickly. There are a lot of angry people out there whom hospitals and doctors are only dimly aware of. You can, of course, treat the medical side of the illness, but if you fail to address the emotional or psychological side, you will never cure more than 50 per cent of the afflicted patient."

By now you should be exclaiming "but all these patient narratives are by journalists". Yes, that's rather the point. If you are intelligent, educated and articulate, you stand a better than average chance of being listened to. Or, if a journalist, of getting published. But my patients on the Bellingham estate are no less human and no less immersed in their own subjective worlds. Should I not attempt to value and to decode their narratives also?

Listening and talking

One cannot offer listening as a panacea without reflecting on what listening actually means. Listening requires:

- Giving the patient the space and the time to express themselves.
- Attending to what the patient is actually saying (as opposed to what you would like them to say).
- Helping the patient to overcome barriers to disclosure.
- Valuing the patient's contribution as the equal of one's own.
- Having the knowledge of the broader world, and the skills to process what the patient says, to gain some insight into the patient's world.

There has been a healthy emphasis recently on valuing the patient as a partner in health care.[14] This has come from the GP Committee of the BMA (the Doctor–Patient Partnership), the RCGP,[15] and from the government.[16] In my own area of South London new models of community involvement are being pioneered.[17] Listening will have a price tag attached to it.[18] But I say it offers excellent value for money.

Conclusion

Becoming a patient is a frightening experience. Being a patient requires a high level of mental and emotional activity that may be invisible to doctors unless we recognise the language of the patient's world. We all experience life as a narrative. As doctors we face a choice. Do we conquer the patient's narrative, forcing it to labour for the project of medicine. Or do we accept a role as the patient's assistant, seeking to help the patient to create their life, helping them with the imperfections and difficulties posed by pathology along the way?

References

1 Carr-Brion J, 1995. Learning to live with the label of psychiatric illness. Personal View. BMJ; 311: 1511–2.
2 Reichenberg F, 1996. Both sides of the coin. Personal View. BMJ; 312: 982.
3 Benbow S, 1995. Is it worth it? Personal View. BMJ; 311: 1511.
4 Davis P, 1992. On the other side of the tracks. Personal View. BMJ; 304: 126–7.
5 LaCombe M, ed., 2000. On Being a Doctor "Voices of Physicians and Patients". Philedelphia: Americal College of Physicians.
6 McCormick A et al, 1995. Who sees their general practitioner and for what reason? Health Trends; 27 (2): 34–5.
7 Brody H, 1992. The healer's power. New Haven: Yale University Press. Chapter 1.
8 Moos R and Schaefer J, 1984. The crisis of physical illness: an overview and conceptual approach. Chapter 1 in Moos R (ed.) Coping with physical illness; Vol 2: New Perspectives. New York: Plenum.
9 Kubler Ross E, 1969. On death and dying. New York: Macmillan.
10 von Neumann J and Morgenstern O, 1953. Theory of games and economic behaviour. New York: Wiley.
11 Torrance G, 1976. Social preferences for health states: an empirical evaluation of three

measurement techniques. Socio-Economic Planning Sciences; 10: 129–36.

12 Smeeth L, 2000. Commentary: patients, preference, and evidence. BMJ; 320: 1384.

13 Beauchamp T and Childress J, 1994. Principles of biomedical ethics. 4th edition. Oxford: Oxford University Press: Chapter 5.

14 Coulter A, 1999. Paternalism or partnership? Editorial. BNJ; 319: 719–20.

15 Williamson C, 1998. The rise of doctor–patient working groups. BMJ; 317: 1374–7.

16 Department of Health, 1999. Patient and public involvement in the new NHS. London: HMSO.

17 Fisher B, Neve H and Heritage Z, 1999. Community development, user involvement, and primary health care. BMJ 18: 749–50.

18 Mariotto A, 1999. Patient partnership is not a magic formula. Letter. BMJ; 319: 783.

5 Psychological models

Medicine is not only a science; it is also an art. It does not consist of compounding pills and plasters; it deals with the very processes of life, which must be understood before they may be guided.

Paracelsus (c.1493–1541) Swiss physician and alchemist

Die grosse Wundarznei

Ideas are much easier to believe if they are comforting... Just as we swallow food because we like it not because of its nutritional content, so do we swallow ideas because we like them and not because of their rational content.

Richard Asher, Talking Sense

A merry heart doeth good like a medicine.

Proverbs Ch17 v22

Chapter summary

There are psychological models of health and health-related behaviour. These explain part of a patient's experience of illness and of a doctor's experience of treating patients and some of the problems that arise in this process.

Introduction

If there is more to medicine than biology then what is the rest made of? It is made of thoughts. The doctor's thoughts and, more importantly, the patient's thoughts. Thoughts, and the belief systems from which they arise, are more complex and more substantial than we might think.

Remember the thesis of Chapter 2: that the only world we know is the model we make of it? To repeat Wittgenstein: "The world is the totality of facts, not of things." We cannot dismiss thoughts and beliefs as insubstantial. They themselves are our world.

The next few chapters look at what we know about the patient's world from a number of different perspectives. But which of these perspectives is true? To some extent they all are. They each show a piece of a whole picture, from a particular point of view. If doctors have a professional "gaze" then so do psychologists, sociologists and anthropologists. They all map out the world as seen from their individual, but restricted, gaze. If we add together their individual contributions, like adding together the political, topographical and geological maps in an atlas, then gradually we can arrive at a fuller picture of the whole. The more we understand of this complex game called medicine the more we are likely to avoid harm, and sometimes do some good.

What contribution does Psychology bring to this whole picture, and what is the territory of its gaze? Health Psychology examines individual beliefs and behaviours, and seeks to describe the links between them.

On the first day of medical school you might have believed this:

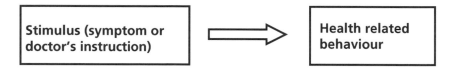

But people are not automata. There's lots going on in that central arrow linking the two boxes. And that means sometimes the arrow doesn't point in what we think is the right direction at all.

This chapter talks a lot about "health behaviours". This means any behaviour that is related to health or affecting health outcomes, such as:

- Smoking, or trying to stop smoking.
- Deciding whether to ignore a symptom, self-treat or see a doctor.
- Attending/not attending a screening procedure such as a cervical smear.
- Complying or not complying with medication.

This chapter looks firstly at some individual thought processes described in the literature. The second part of the chapter examines how such thought processes affect health behaviours.

How do we think?

Making sense

Schon has described the huge indeterminacy present in the world.[1] The swamp of uncertainty that surrounds much of our lives. We may wish to stick to the high ground where facts seem clearer, but most of real life happens in the swamp. But to live our lives without some sense of structure is both intolerable and impossible. Scientifically we cannot prove that the sun will rise tomorrow, but we prefer to live our lives on the assumption that it will.

There is therefore a human need to make sense of everyday events. To create a framework of meaning and causality. The framework doesn't have to be scientifically valid (much less "true"), but it does need to work for us, as a day-to-day explanatory model.

Press cutting

Catford and Hither Green Newsreel, June 1999. p 10.

Mercury Personal Communications has been given conditional planning permission for the building of a base station with mast and associated cabin on land at Hither Green Sidings, Lee [South London] …

Earlier, 149 people had signed a petition objecting to the proposal. One ground for objection was "the health risk including the possible link to cancer". Another ground was that children's future schooling and family plans had been upset, and one person had suffered from nervous tension and had had to seek medication from a doctor.

It is easy for us to rubbish such examples of everyday belief systems as "unscientific", but this is to ignore the function and focus of such models. (It also ignores the ephemeral and provisional nature of scientific beliefs themselves.) This press cutting illustrates what occurs when the public sails into an area of the common folk map labelled "Here be dragons". The area is inadequately explored and processed within the common belief system. But before writing off the map for having such a label we should notice what this model achieves.

This press cutting illustrates one item that lies outside the boundary of a contemporary urban folk model. "Here be dragons" may also encompass the dangers of radiation, genetically modified foods, BSE, mobile phones, aspartame, cloning, etc. (The border may be re-drawn at short notice, for example to exclude MMR vaccine.) But what lies inside the "terra cognito" of such a folk map? Inside we will find some sort of norms about social interaction, childcare, daily living, work, relationships, shopping and hundreds of other mundane life skills. These skills are complex and important. The map gives a common accepted structure to shared life needs.

People prioritise their learning to generate a version of the real world that serves their particular needs. Pure Darwin. The fact that a scientific analysis of the risk–benefit profile of telephone masts does not lie within their priority area for exploration and mapping does not show that their personal map doesn't work – quite the contrary. It shows that their mapping system focuses on their everyday operational needs, and doesn't waste time on things they don't need to know. Acceptance of peripheral novelties into the mapped area could be a threat. Western technology has given us Thalidomide, landmines, nuclear fallout, BSE, answerphones, techno-classic music and personalised junk mail – suspicion is an appropriate adaptive reaction to novelty.

These personal belief maps may therefore lack scientific validity, but they are appropriate to the needs of their owners. What do we know of how they work? Let us first look at a number of basic themes that explain the apparent irrationality of lay health beliefs and behaviour. We shall find that "irrational" beliefs are in fact "other-rational" – they are rational within lay models that are

Symptoms: My back suddenly hurts – I have back pain.

Perceived cause: It started after decorating the ceiling yesterday, therefore:

> 1 I must have pulled a muscle.
> 2 I must have slipped a disc.
> 3 The window was open and it was cold – I must have caught a chill.
> 4. I must be getting unfit.
> 5 I'm getting old – it must be arthritis.

Time line: for 1, 3 and 4 – "This will last a couple of days."

> for 2 – "I'll be laid up for weeks."
> for 5 – "I might have this pain for the rest of my life."

Consequences: for 1 and 3 – "I'll miss the match on Saturday."

> for 2 and 5 – "I might lose my job."
> for 4 – "I'm going to have to get fit again."
> for any – "I can't do the shopping – I'm going to have to cope without being able to bend over – I can't see my friends – I'm going to need to get some painkillers."

Curability/controllability:

> for any – "If I rest it will get better."
> "If I exercise it will get better."
> "If I go to the doctor s/he will make it better."
> "There's not much anyone can do."

Leventhal therefore demonstrates that the consequence of an illness relies as much on what is going on in the patient's head as on what is going on in their body.

Making sense = control

With a single common symptom there is a branching pathway of beliefs that will determine how the patient reacts to his illness, and what his expectations from medical intervention may be.

These possibilities share some things in common. They all:

- give the patient an explanatory framework;
- help them to devise coping strategies (which may or may not be appropriate from a medical perspective);
- help them to guard against further threats to their health and decide whether to seek help.

This system of beliefs therefore may or may not be "medically accurate". However it does give the patient the ability to understand, to cope and to plan. Given the lack of benefit from medical intervention for back pain the patients' illness beliefs are therefore much more important than the doctor's "diagnosis" in this situation.

Patients are not passive. Patients cope with most illness without medical intervention. Even where medical intervention is needed (or sought anyway) patients still do most of the mental work involved in coping with the illness. Making sense is part of keeping or taking back a sense of control. This is one of the patient's most important psychological tasks in illness.

Other people get ill

Illness beliefs are essential tools for survival in the face of illness. However, some mechanisms overprotect a person from the psychological threat of illness and so reduce their ability to deal with illness realistically. This is an example of the ego-defence mechanism of denial.

Weinstein asked subjects to rate their risk of getting specific health problems in comparison to other people of the same age and sex.[5] Most people rated their risk as lower than average. As not everyone can be less likely than average to contract an illness he labelled this phenomenon "unrealistic optimism". Other people get ill.

Weinstein identifies four cognitive factors that worked to create unrealistic optimism:

- Lack of personal experience of the problem leading to a belief that any threat must be distant.
- Belief that the individual is somehow able to prevent the problem.
- The belief that as the problem has not happened so far it must be unlikely to happen in the future.
- The belief that the problem is more unusual than it really is.

Weinstein argues that people show a selective focus when considering risk. People frame their perception of risk depending on the conclusion they are inclined to make. When considering the risk to themselves they become the optimist whose glass is half full, when considering the risk to others they are the pessimist whose glass is half empty. "I won't get lung cancer – I only smoke ten a day" is seen as compatible with "He's a smoker, so now he's got lung cancer".

One could think of this mechanism as part of a "lay gaze", to parallel the concept of the doctor's gaze described by Foucault.[6] In both the lay and the doctor's gaze the perspective is distorted in order to reinforce the observer's view of the world, and the primacy of one's own place within it. It makes for a smoother ride through life; and what the heck – it often works.

Locus of control

One of the first things I was taught as a student was to differentiate between the "ever present" and the "never present". The ever present are patients who cannot sneeze without asking your advice. Their notes contain more information than the EU regulations on the import of butter. The never present would reduce their own dislocated shoulder by referring to a Clint Eastwood film. Their records could be sent airmail. If one day they actually ring up then you'd better get round there quick with a defibrillator.

There are many factors that affect the decision to see the doctor, such as the burden of actual physical disease, learned behaviour, stress and lack of social support. One big factor within the individual is the "locus of control" (LOC). Some people tend to see events that affect them as being largely or potentially within their control. Others see themselves more as a passive observer of events that, although affecting them, remain outside their control. Wallston describes the first group as having an internal locus of control, the second as having an external locus of control.[7] The locus of control for this second group may lie either in "powerful others" (such as a doctor, or "the council") or in the hands of fate.

A patient's locus of control may have a powerful effect on their health-related behaviour. A doctor may tell three patients that they have problem X, and receive three different responses:

Linked case reports – three diabetics

Frank is a retired engineer. On being diagnosed diabetic he grabbed all the literature on offer and promptly joined the BDA. You now see him twice a year. He has lost weight, monitors his blood sugars and runs a HbA1 of 6.8% on diet alone.

LOC: Internal

Cognitive assumption: "What should I do to control my problem?"

Betty is a middle-aged clerk. She has been diabetic for a few years, and has become one of your heartsink patients. Her body mass index hovers around 40, and her HbA1 and frequency of attendance are both too large for your comfort. Whatever oral medication you give her causes side effects, her diet "doesn't work" and you contemplate gloomily the inevitable storms ahead if you start her on insulin. Not to mention that the glycosuria of her poor diabetic control is probably the only thing that stops her BMI catching up with her age.

LOC: External i. = Powerful other

Cognitive assumption: "What will you do to cure my problem?"

John is unemployed and in his late thirties. He is obese, and had the misfortune to have his diabetes initially precipitated by a two week course of prednisolone prescribed for his unstable asthma. He is on oral medication, but the computer record suggests that he gets a two month supply about every four or five months. He defaults from follow-up, and when you finally manage to nail him down for an annual review he receives your comments on his results with the same wan smile that he normally reserves for your advice about diet and compliance with medication.

LOC: External ii. = Fate

Cognitive assumption: "Que sera sera" (It's not my fault and I don't expect your treatment will be much use so there's not much point taking it anyway.)

What these cases also illustrate is that LOC is not just an abstruse theoretical notion. It is a major factor in determining the health outcomes in real patients. It is just as important a factor as any biomedical indicator. There are ways of measuring LOC, and these measures have been shown to predict health-related behaviours.[8]

Locus of control is not set in stone: it may vary according to the situation. I might have an internal LOC for dealing with stress and an external LOC for dealing with a car breakdown. It's not always simple to categorise – making a commitment to follow the doctor's advice can be an example of internal LOC.

LOC will also depend on how challenging I perceive a problem to be, and how many other problems I am facing at the same time. I may generally have an internal LOC, but a major threat such as bereavement, even if there are no technical problems I couldn't deal with myself, may exceed my coping capacity. I may need to partition off some of my problem and lend it to someone else for a while. Or if I am already coping successfully with five ongoing problems, the sixth might be the final straw and make me want to offload one or two elsewhere. Even though LOC is a model with problems it is still a helpful model for understanding behaviour within the consultation.

Self-efficacy

This is not so much a way of thinking as a cognitive variable, analogous perhaps to IQ (and similar to it as an idea that feels right but is difficult to validate).

Schwarzer sees self-efficacy as the belief that one is able to control and to change one's own behaviour.[9] It is similar to Ajzen's concept of "perceived behavioural control",[10] and to what Kobasa calls "hardiness".[11]

Kobasa attributes three elements to hardiness:

- **Control:** a belief in one's ability to act in the face of stress.
- **Commitment:** a sense of involvement and meaning in work, values and relationships.
- **Challenge:** an expectation that demanding and stressful situations will be successfully overcome.

It is interesting that three psychologists have independently created such similar constructs, similar also to the common-sense notions of willpower and positive thinking. This suggests to me that there is a worthwhile category floating about there somewhere, but that it has not yet been clearly enough understood or defined.

The idea of self-efficacy or hardiness is important, even if it is poorly defined. It has been shown repeatedly to be one of the strongest predictors of patients' actual (as opposed to intended) health-related behaviours. Beck and Lund showed that self-efficacy was a stronger determinant of persistence with dental flossing than the level of fear of dental disease.[12] Wurtele and Maddux found that self-efficacy was more important than external persuasion for participating in regular exercise.[13] Maddux and Rogers found that self-efficacy was more important than information on the dangers of smoking for those who are trying to quit.[14]

So we don't know what willpower is, but we know it's important. It is a stronger force for behavioural change than anything we can throw at our patients. If we are trying to change behaviour, somehow we must tap into it, and talk it up if we can. It looks like Norman Vincent Peale's approach in *The Power of Positive Thinking* may be more important than we thought.[15]

Thinking about risk

Doctors know a lot about risk. If John Smith is a smoker aged 70 with a BP of 142/85 and a normal cholesterol, then we know:

- He has a 25–30% risk of a cardiovascular event (CVD event) over the next 5 years.[16]
- Medical treatment will reduce his risk of a CVD event by 9% over 5 years. That, of course, is a 9% relative risk reduction, not 9% taken off his 25–30% absolute risk.

(We also know that if John Smith never saw a doctor, but simply stopped smoking, his risk would fall to 15–20%, a much more impressive health gain, but a different story.)

So doctors have a model of risk that is based on mathematics, and which uses measures such as:

Absolute risk: There is a 25–30% probability of John Smith having a CVD event in 5 years.

Relative risk: John Smith is 1.6 times as likely to have a CVD event in the next 5 years as his identical but non-smoking twin brother.

Number Needed to Treat (NNT): We would have to treat 11 John Smiths for 5 years to prevent one CVD event.

Such risk models are a powerful tool for making judgements about the biomedical significance of medical conditions, and the biomedical effectiveness of possible interventions. Mathematical models, together with evidence from randomised controlled trials (RCTs), form the basis for the current drive towards "evidence-based medicine".

Patients also know a lot about risk. The trouble is that, except for the few patients with a scientific training, the models of risk used bear little relation to the mathematical risk models used by doctors. Davison found that the lay classification of risk is based on a polarity model rather than the gradation of a continuing spectrum.[17] You are either "high risk" or "low risk". This model identifies "likely candidates" for illness. Thus a beer-swilling, heavy-smoking overweight man would (rightly) be seen as at high risk of a heart attack. But if he doesn't have a heart attack and his healthy living neighbour does, this is not seen as an artefact of a small sample within a large complex graduated risk model. It is seen instead as evidence that any sort of risk model is unreliable (the "my father smoked sixty a day until he was 97" effect known so well to all health workers).

One might ask why there is a lay notion of high risk versus low risk at all if this same classification is seen as scarcely worth the paper it's not written on. Davison found that there is a second element in the lay risk model. He found that three other factors were perceived to determine health outcomes. These three were luck, fate and destiny: big forces outside my control but which determine my future.

If for one rationalist moment you doubt the reality of these ideas in popular thinking, just consider how the National Lottery and other similar low-chance gambols are advertised. "There's a one in 20 million chance it could be you"? No way. Rather: "It could be you, so cross your fingers to boost your luck." Or the picture of "Lady Luck" smiling at you from Mount Olympus. It has been said that the National Lottery is a tax for the mathematically challenged. I think it just demonstrates that lay models of probability are not based on maths, but upon an innate sense of personal significance within the universe. Sort of existential ideas of reference.

So a lay model of risk could be understood to function like this:

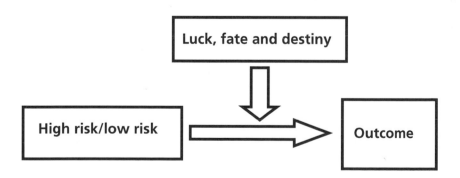

As I am a doctor I've probably written this section with an amused and patronising tone. After all, I know my mathematical models are a much better way of predicting which groups are at risk of illness. I think though that this misses the point. John Smith is not the slightest bit interested which group is at risk. He wants to know if he is going to have a heart attack. *And we cannot tell him!* My job as a doctor is to predict the proportion of my patient list that will get ill, and maybe reducing that figure a little. John Smith's job, as a specialist in being John Smith, is to plan his life according to what suits and what bothers him. And my mathematical model doesn't give him the individual answer that he needs. If we are not talking populations but talking individuals then it comes down to "Do I or don't I take action X?" Suddenly a nice high risk/low risk model looks like a better fit.

Where the model doesn't serve individuals well is in its potential for media manipulation. The "Jaws effect" – (who goes sea swimming after watching "Jaws"?). In 1995 the Committee on Safety of Medicines reported that third generation combined oral contraceptives carried double the risk of venous thromboembolism (VTE) of older COCs.[18] This was widely reported in the press, with little regard for the fact that the actual figures were for an increase of VTE from 15 to 30 per 100,000 women per year, with a death rate of 3 per million women per year. (Again the problem is that relative risk figures are meaningless without reference to the absolute risk.) This led to a pill scare with thousands of women giving up the pill, despite there being a 0.0000033% chance of death. The tragedy was a measurable rise in unwanted pregnancy. The irony is that these women exchanged a 3 per million chance of death from VTE on 3rd generation COCs for a 6 per million chance of death from VTE in pregnancy. Still there were thousands of extra papers sold, so that's all right then, isn't it?

If our risk models come from different planets, is it possible for doctors and patients to talk to one another about risk at all? This is a big question with no easy answers.[19]

The mathematical risk model itself has its difficulties. A major difficulty is the effects of framing on how the questions are asked. Framing is the "spin" we put onto facts. "Would you take a treatment that will reduce your risk of a stroke by 45%?" may be the same question as "would you take a drug that had a 97% probability of doing no you good?" And yet it might be likely to produce a different answer.[20] This is because it is drawing on different parts of a medical model of risk: the relative risk reduction and the NNT respectively. Misselbrook and Armstrong showed that by choosing a particular perspective one can profoundly influence the answers.[21] Far from giving choice, therefore, the mathematical model leaves the choice of risk model still in the hands of doctors. Giving the figures for the three different basic ways of expressing risk is likely to confuse, as this is very much "our" territory, "our" planet.

Framing effects measurably influence patients' choices between different health interventions.[22,23] Patients are not alone in being affected by framing. Framing effects have a similarly potent effect on doctors' decisions to treat.[24] Doctors and patients may be equally prone to cognitive bias by choosing from options defined in terms of relative, rather than absolute, risk reduction figures.[25]

Research work has been done to try to quantify the undesirability to patients of different possible risks of illness. One tool is the "Standard Gamble", which balances the negative utility of a particular outcome against a risk of sudden death.[26] Another is the "Time Trade-off", which values improvements in health status by comparing them to the amount of life expectancy an individual is prepared to forgo to achieve them.[27] The problem is that these are not modelled from the real choices that face patients. They cannot answer the burning question of "do you think it worthwhile taking bendrofluazide for 20 years when it probably won't actually change what happens to me?"

Sir Kenneth Calman, the then Chief Medical Officer, made a brave attempt to cross the patient–doctor divide in 1996. In the introduction to his annual report "On the State of the Public Health 1995" he highlighted the problems of "the language of risk" as one of five public health topics "of particular importance". It is worth reviewing his analysis:

Literature review

Calman K. On the State of the Public Health 1995. London: HMSO, 1996. Introduction.

Calman observes that there is no vocabulary for risk that is common to doctors and patients. Individuals make paradoxical choices due to problems conceptualising risk, e.g. stopping the pill due to a pill scare (minute risk), whilst continuing to smoke (much greater risk). Different people choose differently when faced with the same risk information. Calman proposes a new classification for risk:

Negligible: an adverse event occurring at a frequency below 1 in a million, e.g. death by lightning strike.

Minimal: an adverse event occurring in the range between 1 in a million and 1 in 100,000, e.g. death in a railway accident.

Very low: a risk of between 1 in 100,000 and 1 in 10,000, e.g. death from leukaemia.

Low: a risk of between 1 in 10,000 and 1 in 1,000, e.g. death due to RTA.

Moderate: a risk of between 1 in 1,000 and 1 in 100, e.g. death from smoking 10 cigarettes per day.

High: a risk greater than 1 in 100, e.g. gastrointestinal side effects from antibiotics.

Calman expresses his hope that the public can become full partners in the process of risk assessment.

It seems unlikely that Calman's definition of "high risk" as being a risk of >1% would correspond to the bimodal lay concept of high risk. Calman's hope is that if we all talk about risk more we may eventually arrive at a shared vocabulary. This is a noble hope, but with large conceptual hurdles to be overcome.

In the meantime we must make interplanetary communication as best we can. It is possible to translate risk speak into lay speak if we try.[28] We need to beware of harming patients through untranslated doctor speak. Marteau gives the example of the harm that can be caused by raising personal perceptions of vulnerability to disease through screening.[29] We need to beware the pitfalls of relative risk. Chatellier usefully exhorts us to use NNT as our chief risk model when considering the needs of the individual patient.[30] This can be translated into the "personal probability of benefit" (PPB) in order to relate a treatment benefit as meaningfully as possible to the individual. (PPB = 1/NNT, multiplied by 100 to express as a percentage, i.e. an intervention with an NNT of 7 gives a PPB of 14%.)

Summary

Medical training transforms our thought processes, suiting them to the task of making medical decisions appropriate to populations. Outside of medicine, the process of living develops patients' thought processes to equip them to make decisions appropriate to their individual interests within a world of huge uncertainty. Both worlds are appropriate to the survival needs of the individuals within them. Any overlap of these two worlds is problematic.

Health beliefs

Consultation report

Dr Biotech is a busy GP in his 40s. Mrs Stereotype is a widow in her 70s.

Dr B: Hello, have a seat, what seems to be the problem?

Mrs S: Doctor, can you give me some laxatives? It's my constipation you see.

Dr B: Tell me about your constipation...

Mrs S: Oh, well, I've always been constipated. My Fred always said it was the London water. I'm so sorry to trouble you with it, but it's giving me such headaches when the poison builds up in my system. The poison killed my Fred in the end. I've always managed it myself with Finnon Salts and Sennokot every day, and of course I take the Dieselgistics for the headaches, but it's just not helping.

Dr B establishes that the constipation is of gradual onset over 5 years, since Mrs S was started on a repeat scrip for frusemide after an episode of oedema precipitated by a two week course of NSAIDs for OA knees. She has a low-fibre highly refined high-meat-plus-bread-and-jam diet. She has no weight loss, no pain, and passes no blood. Abdominal and PR examination are normal.

> Dr B: Well, I'm glad to say it's not serious. I think we can improve things here, and I'd like to explain what we need to do. First I want you to stop the Frusemide and the Co-proxamol as I think they may be making matters worse.
>
> Mrs S: But Doctor, I never used to pass enough water without the Frusemide. When I forgot one last month I didn't pass half as much water that morning.
>
> Dr B: No no, it really doesn't matter how much water you pass. The second thing is that I want you to start a high-fibre, high-fluid diet. You must have less fry-ups, less meat and eggs, but more bran products.
>
> Mrs S: But I've always eaten well, Doctor. My mother always made sure we had lots of good food to build us up. She said we needed meat to make us strong, and she was always prepared to spend a little bit more to get us white bread and jam. I was one of seven, and my mother never lost any of us.
>
> Dr B: No no, that's all wrong. Look, I'll give you this up-to-date booklet that will explain what you ought to be eating, and come and see me again in a month.

Is there a problem with this consultation? Dr B explored the problem and made an accurate diagnosis. He produced a good management plan of action that he explained, and gave written information. He avoided the temptation to give in and give laxatives. Surely the problem is Mrs S? She seems quite stubborn, and holds all sorts of weird beliefs. She doesn't seem to realise that Dr B is the expert here, with nine years of medical training.

Thinking like this may make us feel more clever than our patients, and even lend us a kind of moral superiority. It is also rather futile. Are there any more constructive ways of approaching this type of problem? Finding out the patient's health beliefs and understanding their proper function gives us another way of looking at these issues.

Reaction to illness (or symptoms which may or may not mean illness) is not set as a biological inevitability or instinct. It is based on patients' reactions to the beliefs they hold about the nature and consequences of the symptoms. These beliefs are not straightforward, and only partly coincide with bio-medical models of illness. They are influenced also by social and cultural factors. Thus they are not obvious. Patients have often learned that doctors do not value their health beliefs, and so they are commonly reluctant to discuss them. Also patients may believe that their health beliefs spring directly from a 'biological reality' and so feel that discussion is frivolous. This is reinforced by the fact that health beliefs often derive from personal anecdotal experience (just as do many beliefs of doctors) and will therefore be strongly held. Our models of the way things are rely heavily on our own experience.

Health beliefs also exist within cultural norms. They affect the symptoms a patient complains of. A hassled parent with a grumpy boss in the UK may present with headaches, whilst their *alter ego* from Africa may present with a sensation of "pains all over" and their colleague from Asia with "burning all over". Health beliefs demonstrate another facet of mind/body unity.

The making of worlds

Let us consider the belief world a doctor manufactures when the elderly patient comes complaining of constipation. Dr B has never seen Mrs S's colon, but he has a model of it in his mind. That model encompasses the structure and function of the bowel, and the things that may affect it. That model is based on pictures from textbooks, dissection, Surgical Housemanship, X-rays, opinions passed on from "experts", his experience of patients, and his experience of his own and his family's bowels. Many of the parts of this model will have evidence to back them up, but perhaps the only evidence that he could actually quote to you would be the evidence of his own experience. The operations and X-rays he has seen, his own experience as a medic, and what affects his own bowels.

Mrs S also comes to the consultation with a model of her colon. Like Dr B, that model encompasses the structure and function of the bowel, and the things that may affect it. It is based on information handed down from her mother, her mother's pharmacist, biology lessons in 1935, her *Encyclopaedia of Family Health* (1950 edition), her broader family and network of neighbours and friends. She too can quote you evidence: her Fred's illness and death; her mother's self-evident success in raising herself and her six siblings; her own headaches; and the obvious benefit she derives from diuretics. This model will also be driven by concerns about the significance of the symptoms she is experiencing. The fact that she has consulted you may mean that she is unable to place all of her symptomatology within her own explanatory map. Her experience therefore comes within the anxious area marked "Here be dragons".

So what happens when two conflicting models meet? Suppose you are a Protestant and I am a Roman Catholic. We meet for ten minutes and I say "No no no, you should be a Catholic." Will my approach work? Does my approach value your own personal journey, and take into account the deep cultural and experiential roots of your beliefs? Would my approach perhaps work if I had a degree in theology? Of course not.

Health beliefs work in a similar way. They will have roots and connections with the broader range of personal and socially related ideas that make up each individual's world. It is naive for us to think that we can "overwrite" our patients' health beliefs with our own, just because we have "MB" after our name. It's not how people work.

So what?

These beliefs have value. They have enabled the patient to understand and deal with their problem up to now. Whilst they could be analysed as "right" or "wrong" according to current medical orthodoxy, this is of no help to your patient. (Does current medical orthodoxy always have that long a shelf life anyway? I was taught that asthma is an emotional problem, never to give β-blockers in LVF, that babies should never be laid on their back, that schizophrenia is caused by dysfunctional parenting...)

Patients' health beliefs have value for two reasons:

- Patients and their families deal with most symptoms and illnesses without seeing a doctor. Fry states that three-quarters of health issues are dealt with within a lay setting.[31] Zola goes further and states that "Virtually every day of our lives we are subject to a vast array of bodily discomforts. Only an infinitesimal amount of these get to a physician".[32] Banks et al found that for every episode of chest pain brought to the doctor 14 chest pains were not brought.[33] Every backache seen in surgery represents 52 backaches that are not seen. And remarkably every episode of loss of energy seen in surgery represents 456 episodes not seen. Lay health beliefs are the appropriate way for the majority of symptoms and minor illnesses to be dealt with. Lay beliefs do not need to be overwritten by medical thinking any more than General Practice medicine needs to be overwritten by hospital medicine. All three are complementary parts of society's coping system. Lay health beliefs deserve our respect.
- When the lay system proves inadequate and a person becomes a patient they still do much of the work. They have to perform many health-related behaviours such as attending appointments, making arrangements for their work and life, taking medications and above all coping with the threat of illness. They cannot suddenly jump into a new cognitive model. They have to do all these things as the people they are. Our job is to support them rather than correct them.

Hothouse or jungle?

Wandering through Kew Gardens is a different experience from finding your way through the jungle. At Kew a tiny proportion of the plant kingdom has been selected, studied and laid out under our control. In the jungle there is a chaotic profusion of life without visible limits. It surrounds. It overwhelms. There are different rules for those who would work in the jungle.

Much of medicine's knowledge base derives from the hothouses of the hospital and the laboratory. General Practice happens in the more challenging and exciting environment of the jungle. We are the naturalists of the streets and homes of our bizarre and tangled jungle of a world. To survive we must observe, we must explore. We must understand how the jungle works.

Sometimes patients' health beliefs seem strange to us.

Consultation excerpt

> Self: I've got your ear swab results. It's growing a funny bug called Pseudomonas. I wonder where that came from? [Meaning "It's not the bug I was expecting."]
>
> Patient (78-yr-old man): I wonder if I picked it up when I was buried in Egypt during the war?

But why should this flight of association seem strange to us? The patient was just joining in our game. I said the bug was unusual. We make associations that at face value are just as strange. A patient complains of being short of breath and we ask if their ankles swell. They complain of tiredness and we ask if they pass more water. Before giving them ibuprofen for their backache we ask if they have asthma. And why should the patient know which "funny bugs" might or might not be quiescent? Last year I probably told his brother-in-law that his shingles was due to the chicken pox virus "lying dormant in your spinal cord since you were a kid".

Given that symptoms are commonplace, taking them to the doctor by definition depends on some interpretative activity, otherwise most of our patients would come to see us on most days. The interpretation of symptoms cannot be done without the guidance of health beliefs.[34] Health beliefs therefore play a central part in the decision whether to see a doctor or to cope within a lay model.

Health beliefs are often the key to what is going on in a consultation.

Consultation excerpt

> Patient (68-yr-old hypertensive woman, widowed one year ago): I have a strange fluttering feeling in my left thigh... [On examination nad, sounds like minor benign fasciculation.]
>
> Self: You look a bit worried by it.
>
> Patient: I was wondering if it was a clot. [*Reassurance that there is no sign of a clot.*]
>
> Patient: I'm more anxious now I'm alone.

What this patient said interested me for a number of reasons. First, the consultation would have missed the point had it jumped from examination to reassurance, missing out "I was wondering if it was a clot?" There is nothing exceptional about the symptom itself that, out of an ocean of minor symptoms in the community, it should be taken on an outing to the doctor. The point of the consultation is that the patient's belief about the symptom needed to be addressed. Without identifying that belief and taking it seriously there can be no communication between the medical and lay planets, much less the possibility of reassurance. (How do you feel when the garage mechanic brushes aside your graphic description of the clanking noise coming from the engine and just tells you not to worry about it?)

Second, this particular consultation demonstrates the patient's own awareness of the mechanisms which determine whether any given symptom is brought to the doctor. "I'm more anxious now I'm alone" implies that she is worried I might think that the symptom is too trivial to "bother the doctor with". She offers an explanation for her bringing the symptom along. Being widowed could have a number of influences on her decision to consult, e.g.:

- An increase in her perceived vulnerability to illness, relating to her husband's illness.
- A decreased support network, reducing her ability to cope with minor illness.

Perhaps she tends to an external locus of control, previously looking to her husband, now having to look elsewhere. Being alone and bereft may have reduced her hardiness. I might have completely missed a "ticket of entry" – actually she wants to talk about her grief or her depression.

Has the penny dropped?

Because doctors live on another planet it is not always easy to guess what the patient's health belief or concerns may be:

> **Consultation excerpt**
>
> A woman in her 40s attends with a physiological tremor that has troubled her recently as she has had to perform in front of colleagues. I want to double check that it's not thyroid disease, but I think she looks worried. I know why – I bet she's worried it could be Parkinson's disease.
>
> Self: What did you think might be causing this?
> Patient: I don't know – I haven't the faintest idea.
> Self [*not convinced*]: You look quite worried.
> Patient: [*pause…*] Well, I was wondering if it could be multiple sclerosis.

Health beliefs therefore need to be explored. This is not always easy. We are the "experts", and patients may be worried that we will dismiss their beliefs as foolish. This may be worse with cultural groups (such as the elderly) who perceive doctors as having particular social authority:

The patient is an 87-yr-old widow who seems to me to be "unduly anxious" about minor simple fluid retention secondary to varicose veins.

Self: What do you think it might be?
Patient: I haven't the faintest. [*Explanation of simple fluid retention and suggestions for management.*]

Patient still looks hesitant and anxious, therefore:

Self: You seem worried – tell me about it?
Patient: Do you remember my Arthur? Before he died [*of chronic bronchitis with heart failure*] 10 years ago his ankles swelled.

In the early part of this consultation I perceived the patient to be "unduly anxious". We have a choice as to how we view our patients:

Option 1: patients are thick.
Option 2: patients have a reason for their belief systems, which are therefore rational, in the sense that they form a coherent system.

There are many examples of qualitative research that explore lay health belief systems. In a classic paper entitled "Feed a cold and starve a fever", Cecil Helman, a North London GP, shows how the orthodox medical beliefs of a few generations ago are alive and well in lay belief systems.[35] Interestingly he shows how modern models, such as bacteria and viruses, can be incorporated into lay belief models, and used to strengthen them rather than to change them.

In another classic paper Mildred Blaxter explores lay ideas of disease causation:

Literature review

Blaxter M, 1983. The causes of disease: women talking. Social Science and Medicine; 17, 2: 59–69.

Blaxter talked to 46 working class grandmothers exploring their concepts of disease causation in a semi-structured interview. The diseases the women mentioned included TB, cancer, measles, bronchitis, heart disease, pneumonia, rheumatism, colds and many more.

Disease was conceptualised as a "malevolent entity, residing outside the person, lying in wait to attack". Some diseases such as cancer and TB were often referred to by euphemisms, and were seen as capricious attacks by fate.

There were certain "preferred" categories of causation:

- Infection, e.g. the infectious diseases.
- Heredity and family susceptibility, e.g. bronchitis, arthritis, thrombosis, heart disease, diabetes, meningitis, cancer, tonsillitis.

- Environmental agents, e.g. bronchitis, colds, TB, cancer, pleurisy, Parkinson's disease.
- Stress, e.g. headache, heart disease, thyroid disease, asthma, depression, St Vitus Dance.

Some categories of causation tended to be rejected:

- Natural degenerative processes.
- Idiopathic disease due to random chance.
- Unhealthy behaviours.
- Neglect and poverty.

The common belief by doctors and patients that infections are caused by pathogens is interesting. The women generally called them "germs", and did not divide them into the nice medical categories of bacteria and viruses. It was seen as important to "fight germs", e.g. by the fumigation of rooms and washing clothes in disinfectant.

The womens' models of disease processes were analogous to the medical models that we use, although individual disease explanations will often be very different. The women clearly found their understanding of causation to be an important part of the process of coping with illness.

Blaxter sees the attempt at rational explanation and the importance of understanding the links between life events as common human traits shared by both doctors and patients. It is just the individual elements of our explanatory models that differ; our framework is pretty much the same. But how can a belief system be reasonable if patients do not instantly accept the judgement of the expert? There may be a number of reasons:

- Experts can be wrong. I well remember Mrs L, a charming old lady who called me out on a Sunday afternoon with a worsening of her longstanding burning retrosternal pain which she put down to a particularly heavy Sunday lunch. She seemed perfectly well, and there was nothing to find on examination except minor epigastric tenderness. I increased her Gaviscon and left her some cimetidine. I was of course called back by her husband to confirm her death from a heart attack some two hours later.
- The patient has more at stake than the doctor. If a patient with known diverticular disease attends with a typical attack of diverticulitis I will generally apply Occam's razor and initially diagnose and treat it at face value. "But Doctor, how do you know it's not bowel cancer this time?" Honest answer, "Well I don't". We just call it the management of uncertainty. And yes, I do know about safety netting, but the patient doesn't want to fall off the high wire in the first place.
- The patient's health beliefs may have deep roots in their family network, their culture or their own experience. How can I, as a remote figure they see for 10 minutes three or four times a year, compete with

the rootedness of real-life networks?

- We may lack credibility. We may be too young. When I first joined my current practice some 17 years ago one of the first patients to walk through my door greeted me with the words: "So I'm not seeing the doctor today then?" Or our scientifically correct uncertainty may clash with the patient's need for certainty. I'd been in the practice ten years and I called the Registrar in to see a rash that might have been early Pityriasis rosea in a patient not well known to me. I failed to read the patient's signals, and he turned to me anxiously and asked whether I was fully qualified or "still in training". We may be from the wrong subculture. How can a teenage girl wanting the pill believe that I understand the issues that face her? And what credibility will I have with Mrs L's husband from three paragraphs ago?
- Our objectives may be different from the patient's. An Afro-Caribbean man in his sixties came to see me a couple of weeks ago with a one-year history of gradual-onset loose motions about five times daily. A nice biomedical puzzle to solve. Despite his steady weight and a normal examination I explained to him I would need a couple of blood tests, and would probably want to refer him for a Gastoenterologist's opinion. He then patiently explained to me that he had only come to see me for some antidiarrhoeals so that he could fly without hassle to the Caribbean to attend his brother's funeral.
- We may not always have the patient's interest at heart. I may be prescribing Scragapril instead of the much better drug Ripofopril to stay within my drug budget. And is the doctor really convinced about the safety of MMR, or is he more concerned about his target payments?

Wherever possible we should explore the patient's health beliefs and work with them. Usually our own health beliefs will overlap with the patient's health beliefs:

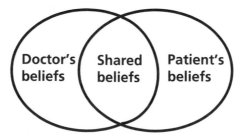

We can then talk up the common ground, and if we want to introduce new ideas or try to modify any of the patient's health beliefs then we can use the shared beliefs as a bridge. Trying to overwrite the patient's beliefs with our own will only teach the patient that we are arrogant and have not listened to them properly.

What if it doesn't work?

There are times when lay health beliefs and medical orthodoxy just don't talk. These tend to make for our most challenging and frustrating consultations. A good example would be the significance of childhood fever.

Literature review

Blumenthal I, 1998. What parents think of fever. Family Practice; 15: 513–16

This is a questionnaire-based study of 392 parents attending a paediatric outpatient department. It aims to explore parents' beliefs about the significance and management of childhood fever. Key findings:

- Two-thirds of parents used thermometers on their children, mostly of the inaccurate liquid crystal type.
- But 91% of parents did not know how to take a child's temperature accurately.
- 24% thought that a temperature of 37° indicates a fever.
- 46% stated that a child with a fever should always be seen by a doctor.
- 27% thought that a child with a fever should always be admitted to hospital for observation.
- Asked what would be the likely outcome if a child's fever was "not treated":
  - 6% said natural recovery
  - 65% said fitting
  - 15% said brain damage
  - 7% said death

As these parents were at a paediatric outpatient department we might expect greater levels of anxiety and a greater experience of serious childhood illness than in the general population. Even so, all of a sudden the anxious tone of all those out-of-hours calls seems a lot more understandable.

So what do we do when our beliefs and the patient's beliefs come from different planets?

- It may be that differing beliefs do not matter. (If diuretics are necessary for hypertension it doesn't matter if a patient takes them because of a belief that they need to pass more water.) It is better to be pragmatic.
- If differing beliefs do matter then the nature of your task is not so much "conversion to orthodoxy", but rather to build a bridge across which you can share the most important ideas and plans. This involves respecting the integrity of both models and "talking up" any shared beliefs. Restructure what you say so that new ideas add to or modify (rather than replace) the patient's existing health belief framework.

- Occasionally there is no shared ground, or it may be inadequate.

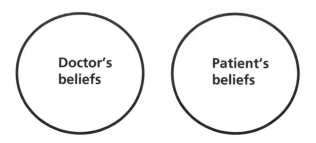

Whatever else we do it is important to see where the beliefs are coming from and to respect the reasons that the patient holds those beliefs, even if we see little merit in the beliefs themselves. Not every consultation has an ideal ending.

The health belief model

This chapter has shown that cognitive processes and health beliefs are an important determinant of health behaviours. In the 1960s Rosenstock formulated a model to describe the relationship between health beliefs and behaviour.[36] This model was modified by Becker in the 1970s, and is known as the Health Belief Model (HBM).[37]

Becker states that health behaviours are not a simple stimulus/response, but that a possible stimulus to a behaviour (such as a symptom, or a health education message) is first processed via the HBM to determine the response.

Again we are faced with the choice of what to think about patients. It is tempting for us to denigrate health behaviours that are not medically approved. Why, for example, don't patients exercise more, when we know that exercise is good for you?

Option 1: patients are thick.
Option 2: patients have a reason for their health behaviours, which are therefore rational and open to understanding and possible modification.

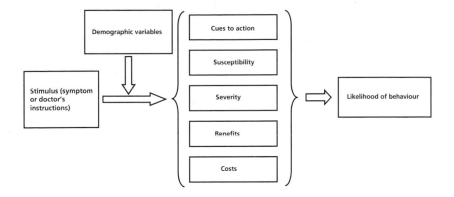

So can the HBM tell us anything useful about why patients do or don't exercise?

Demographic variables: the model acknowledges that issues such as age, ethnicity, gender and income will affect the whole process. There would be more barriers to be overcome for a low-income elderly Asian woman to join a gym than for a young Western male.

Cues to action: Health behaviours do not just happen. I might have a general desire to exercise, but it may be number 27 on my list of priorities, and I'm only juggling up to number 8. A cue to action may make me push a behaviour up the list. Cues to action may be internal ("I really want to go trekking in the Himalayas, I'd better get fit"), or external ("Thank you for the exercise bike, darling, it's just what I need").

Perceived susceptibility to illness: "All my family get heart disease in middle age and I'm getting unfit. I'd better do something about it." Or "None of my workmates exercise and we're all healthy enough. Why should I bother, it's a mug's game."

Perceived severity of the problem: "I've put on a stone in the last ten years – that's not too bad." Or "I've put on a stone in the last ten years – that's gross."

Perceived benefits: "Exercise will make me feel good and look great."

Perceived costs: "Exercise is hard work, I'll have to give up a couple of hours a week, it's a pain getting to the gym and it'll cost me a fortune."

Thus, if we believe exercise is relevant to a patient's health, our role is not to declare: "You need to exercise". Our role is to latch into the patients health belief system and see if there are blocks that can be overcome and positive beliefs that can be built on.

The HBM is really no more than a provisional list of factors which influence a multi-dimensional decision. One could add other factors, such as the effect of ego-defence mechanism such as denial, or the level of motivation present.

It fails to acknowledge that much of what we do is socially determined (but let us leave that for the next chapter). Another big problem is that it does not allow for self-efficacy, which we have already noted as an important predictor of behaviour.

Protection Motivation Theory

Rogers therefore revised the HBM into the Protection Motivation Theory (PMT). This recognises four influences to health-related behaviours:

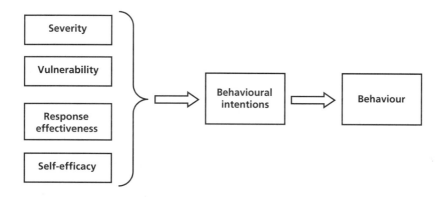

PMT is useful in clearly distinguishing behavioural intentions from actual behaviours. It balances "threat appraisal" (severity, vulnerability and response effectiveness) with "coping appraisal" (self-efficacy).

We can imagine ever more complex and comprehensive models. The basic point is simple. The relation between health stimulus and health behaviour is complex. We can identify many factors that affect it.

We don't prescribe β-blockers to asthmatics "because I'm dealing with your blood pressure at the moment". We use a more sophisticated multi-system model. We need also to let our gaze include psychological factors that should affect our understanding of medical management just as much as any drug contra-indication.

Patients are active

Rollnick et al point out that patients are often ambivalent about health behaviours.[38] If you push someone they obey Newton's First Law and exert force in the opposite direction: what Berne describes as a "Why don't you... Yes but..." game.[39] Akerlind et al found that psychosocial factors were a stronger predictor of return to work than the initial severity of symptoms.[40] Patients are not Pavlovian models who react only to symptom stimuli and doctors' instructions. They actively process both.

Conclusions

Patients do not sit passively experiencing symptoms that they bring unprocessed to the doctor. They do not passively obey the doctor's advice about management. To treat patients as automatons is dumb. It is better to lift the bonnet and understand the action that is going on underneath. We should understand the value and function of patients' lay health beliefs, and seek to work with them. It is smart to negotiate, add information, foster motivation, encourage self-efficacy and talk up healthy options. It's smart to treat patients as active stakeholders in the medical game.

References

1 Schon D, 1995. The reflective practitioner. Aldershot: Arena. Chapter 2.

2 Heider F, 1944. Social perception and interpersonal relations. Psychological Review; 51: 358–74.

3 Kelly H, 1967. Attribution theory in social psychology. In D Levine (ed.), Nebraska Symposium on Motivation. Lincoln NB: University of Nebraska Press: pp 192–238.

4 Leventhal et al, 1980. The common sense representation of illness danger. In Rachman S (ed.), Medical Psychology, vol 2. New York: Pergamon. pp 7–30.

5 Weinstein N, 1984. Why it won't happen to me: perceptions of risk factors and susceptibility. Health Psychology; 3: 431–57.

6 Foucault M, 1963. Naissance de la clinique. Paris: Presses Universitaires de France. Translated, 1976, as "The birth of the clinic". London: Tavistock. Chapter 6.

7 Wallston K and Wallston B, 1982. Who is responsible for your health? The construct of health locus of control. In Sanders G and Suls J (eds), Social psychology of health and illness. Hillsdale, NJ: Lawrence Erlbaum Associates. pp 65–95.

8 Murray M and McMillan C, 1993. Health beliefs, locus of control, emotional control and women's cancer screening behaviour. British Journal of Clinical Psychology; 32: 87–100.

9 Schwartzer R, 1992. Self-efficacy in the adoption and maintainance of health behaviours: Theoretical approaches and a new model. In Self-efficacy: thought control of action. London: Hemisphere.

10 Ajzen I, 1988. Attitudes, personality and behaviour. Milton Keynes: Open University Press.

11 Kobasa S, Maddi S and Puccetti M, 1982. Personality and exercise as buffers in the stress–illness relationship. Journal of Behavioural Medicine; 5: 391–404.

12 Beck K and Lund A 1981. The effects of health threat seriousness and personal efficacy upon intentions and behaviour. Journal of Applied Saocial Psychology; 11: 401–15.

13 Wurtele S and Maddux J 1987. Relative contributions of protection motivation theory components in predicting exercise intentions and behaviour. Health Psychology; 6: 453–66.

14 Maddux J and Rogers R 1983. Protection motivation and self-efficacy: A revised theory of fear appeals and attitude change. Journal of Experimental Social Psychology; 19: 469–79.

15 Peale NV, reissue 1996. The power of positive thinking. Ballantine Books.

16 National Heart Foundation of New Zealand, 1999. Tables, quoted in Clinical Evidence. London: BMJ Publishing Group, Issue 1, June: Appendix 1.

17 Davison C et al, 1991. Lay epidemiology and the prevention paradox: the implications of coronary candidacy for health education. Sociology of Health & Illness; 13, 1: 1–19.

18 Committee on Safety of Medicines, 1995. Combined oral contraceptives and thrombo-embolism. London: Committee on Safety of Medicines.

19 Kee F, 1996. Patients' prerogatives and perceptions of benefit. BMJ; 312: 958–60.

20 MRC Working Party, 1985. MRC trial of treatment of mild hypertension: principal results. BMJ; 291: 97–104.

21 Misselbrook D and Armstrong D, 2001. Patients' responses to risk information about the benefits of treating hypertension. British Journal of General Practice; 51: 276–9.

22 Jou J et al, 1996. An information processing view of framing effects: the role of causal schemas in decision making. Memory and Cognition; 24 (1): 1–15.

23 Percy M et al, 1995. Assessing preferences about the DNR order: does it depend on how you ask? Medical Decision Making; 15 (3): 209–16.

24 Bucher H et al, 1994. Influence of method of reporting study results on decision of physicians to prescribe drugs to lower cholesterol concentration. BMJ; 309: 761–4.

25 Kee F, 1996. Patients' prerogatives and perceptions of benefit. BMJ; 312: 958–60.

26 von Neumann J and Morgenstern O, 1953. Theory of games and economic behaviour. New York: Wiley.

27 Torrance G, 1976. Social preferences for health states: an empirical evaluation of three measurement techniques. Socio-economic Planning Sciences; 10: 129–36.

28 Glasziou P and Irwig L, 1995. An evidence based approach to individualising treatment. BMJ; 311: 1356–9.

29 Marteau T, 1990. Screening in practice: reducing the psychological costs. BMJ; 301: 26–8.

30 Chatellier G et al, 1996. The number needed to treat: a clinically useful nomogram in its proper context. BMJ; 312: 426–9.

31 Fry J, 1993. General practice the facts. Oxford: Radcliffe Medical Press. Chapter 1.

32 Zola I, 1973. Pathways to the doctor – from person to patient. Social Science and Medicine; 7: 677–89.

33 Banks M et al, 1975;. Factors influencing demand for primary medical care in women aged 20–44 years: a preliminary report. International Journal of Epidemiology; 4 (3): 189–95.

34 Pennebaker J, Epstein D, 1983. Implicit psychophysiology: effects of common beliefs and idiosyncratic physiological responses on symptom reporting. Journal of Personality; 51 (3): 468–96.

35 Helman C, 1978. 'Feed a cold, starve a fever': folk models of infection in an English suburban community, and their relation to medical treatment. Cult. Med. Psychiatry; 2: 107–37.

36 Rosenstock I, 1966. Why people use health services. Millbank Memorial Fund Quarterly; 44: 94–124.

37 Becker M, 1974. The health belief model and personal health behaviour. Health Education Monographs; 2: 324–508.

38 Rollnick S, Kinnersley P, Stott N, 1993. Methods of helping patients with behavioural change. BMJ; 307: 188–90.

39 Berne E, 1964. Games people play. London: Penguin.

40 Akerlind I, Hornquist J, Bjurulf P, 1992. Psychological factors in the long-term prognosis of chronic low back pain patients. Journal of Clinical Psychology; 48 (5): 596–605.

6 Sociological models: i The sick role

I wish I really knew what you meant about being sick. Sometimes I felt so bad I could curl up and die, but I had to go on because the kids had to be taken care of and besides, we didn't have the money to spend for the doctor. How could I be sick? How do you know when you're sick anyway? Some people can go to bed most anytime with anything, but most of us can't be sick, even when we need to be.

A patient's experience, quoted by Zola[1]

Employment is Nature's physician and is essential to human happiness.

Galen

Chapter summary

The experience of illness occurs within a cultural setting. This is a key determinant of health seeking, and health care providing, behaviours.

You'll never walk alone

What is normal?

Few behavioural norms are fixed unalterably, irrespective of time or culture. Normal behaviour is mostly socially defined. Behaviour that leads to social approval among a group of Vikings would lead to a lengthy jail sentence in modern suburbia. Normative interaction from the Arsenal terraces will not be welcomed in a concert hall. And it never fails to amaze me how people drive in Worthing.

Norms for illness behaviour are also socially defined. We saw in the last chapter how individual thought processes and beliefs determine illness behaviours, but the social group sets the normative range within which these behaviours happen.

One could see the issue of psychological versus social explanations of health behaviours as an academic border raid. Surely the point is that most health behaviours are complex responses to a mixture of biomedical, psychological and social stimuli which operate both from within the person themselves and from those around them. We shouldn't be afraid of models competing for our attention. Just stack them up together, and use whichever fits best.

If we consider a health behaviour such as the likelihood of attending a doctor's surgery with symptom X then we could express this two-dimensional model of behaviour like this:

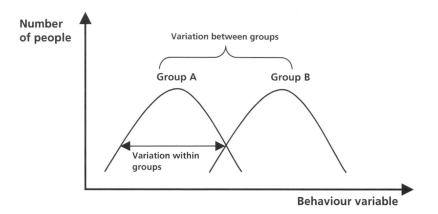

Most variations within a group will be due to psychological variables. Most variations between groups will be due to cultural norms. The behaviour of any given individual depends on both factors.

One can interpret even more of the individual variability of health behaviours within a social framework. Zola's model recognises that, as well as individual health beliefs and a general cultural norm, there may be social "triggers" to the decision to consult:[2]

The occurrence of an interpersonal crisis. It is as if we have a total coping capacity within ourselves. If a crisis removes a source of support, or adds a new strain, then illness that was previously tolerable becomes intolerable. If we ask "Why come now?", the answer often relates to social rather than biomedical factors.

Perceived interference with social or personal relationships. If a problem causes a social disability then its time to see the doctor. Mild acne may be tolerable, but not if there is a new girlfriend in sight.

Perceived interference with vocational or physical activity. A minor leg muscle injury is different for a Premier League footballer than it is for a bank clerk.

Sanctioning. We may be ambivalent about whether a doctor's opinion is needed. Or we may feel foolish about making the decision to consult for ourselves. We may seek support in our decision from family, friends, magazine articles or NHS Direct. There is some evidence for a "lay referral network". In 1960 Friedson proposed that patients consulted doctors after failing to solve their problem via a (possibly extensive) lay network.[3] The idea is that if, say, your partner can't solve the problem you seek someone with more knowledge until you might finally see the doctor. Recently Cornford and Cornford supported this model.[4] They found that 70% of patients with new symptoms reported conversations within their family or social networks that were important in their decision to consult. Men tended to talk to both men and women, but women mainly talked to other women. These conversations were key to symptoms becoming "socially constructed" as illness.

Temporalising of symptoms. "If it's not better by Monday I'll see the doctor." A way of working out if a symptom is self limiting, and setting tolerance boundaries.

The theory of planned behaviour

As the health belief model (HBM) lacks the dimension of social control, Ajzen and Madden developed the theory of planned behaviour:[5]

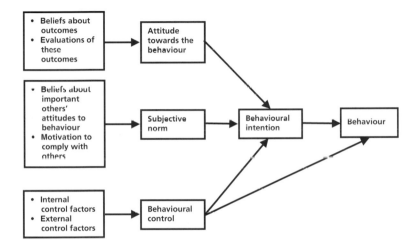

If this looks a bit complicated I would offer a simplified version of Ajzen, like this:

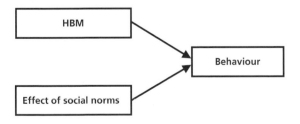

Ajzen's point is that it is meaningless to consider the HBM without considering the effects of social norms.

The sick role

Health behaviours do not stop at the decision to see the doctor/give up smoking/have a smear/take a pill. If the patient believes they are ill then a pattern of behaviours by the patient and by those around them will tend to occur. Parsons called this pattern the sick role.[6] For the sick role to be legitimised socially it must be recognised by a doctor, (e.g. by the giving of a diagnosis and a "sick note"). The doctor performs a key ritual in the rite of passage from person to patient.

The sick role is a syndrome of linked social norms:

The patient is not held to be responsible for his illness. The patient is seen as a victim deserving of help. Others (such as healthcare workers) assume responsibility for fixing the patient's problems.

The patient is temporarily excused from normal social roles. A medical certificate excuses the patient from work/jury service/attendance at court/attendance at an exam, without the penalties which would apply if you didn't turn up because it clashed with your favourite soap opera. More profoundly the sick role may excuse the patient from responsibilities within their family and social network.

The patient must want to get well. The patient must be an unwilling victim, who is seen to want to resume his normal social obligations. This is the main criterion that separates "a patient" from "a malingerer".

The patient must cooperate with the doctor. The doctor acts as the agent of society, first legitimising the patient's entry to the sick role, then guiding him towards the way back out.

Armstrong points out that the sick role thus confers two benefits, and two obligations.[7] The doctor stands as social arbiter to ensure that the benefits and obligations are recognised and legitimised.

If disease = illness = disability then this social arrangement would seem unproblematic. But we have already seen that illness does not wholly correlate with disease. Neither does disability.

The degree of seriousness of disease could be seen to form a continuum from, say, a self-limiting URTI to terminal metastatic cancer. The degree of a patient's disability similarly forms a continuum from the need to spend 30 seconds a day taking a pill, to being completely unable to move, bedbound, and totally reliant on others for every need. The puzzling thing is that there is no simple relationship between the severity of disease within any given diagnosis and the degree of disability experienced by the patient.

Paired case report

Julie Weeks is a 36-year-old mother with chronic back pain. Investigations are non-contributory. She has seen the Rheumatologists who have referred her to the pain clinic. She receives regular certificates as she feels unable to do any sort of work because of pain. I recently completed a medical report for her Orange Badge application.

Gwen Hardy is a 62-year-old widow with moderately severe active rheumatoid arthritis. She has extensive joint damage. She walks slowly with a stick, and drives a specially modified car. She is on methotrexate and attends for regular blood tests. She works full time as an administrator/PA for a boss who has known her for many years. She describes to me what her limitations are at work, and how she has sucessfully negotiated with her boss to find ways round them. When I ask her how she, is she replies, "Oh, very well at the moment, thank you."

So what are we to think about those with relatively low "disease scores" but high "disability scores"? Humans are designed to be problem-solvers. We all have needs to be fulfilled. We have survival needs such as money. We also need recognition and respect. Furthemore we cannot directly enter anyone else's consciousness and compare levels of pain, effort, distress or hardiness. Many life choices are made at an almost subconscious level. Greater levels of disability are found in lower socioeconomic groups, which cannot be accounted for solely by downward social drift due to illness. Some are faced with the choice between a low paid job with hassle and perhaps some discomfort, or the alternative of "disability" with social sanctioning of lessened responsibility and enhanced social benefits. This does not mean that this group are malingerers (although some may be). This is simply to recognise that the sick role is socially sanctioned, and that much of normal behaviour is socially defined.

The trouble is that it is like trying to square the circle. The mixture of social and biomedical models is fraught with difficulty. It is doomed to inconsistency as shown in the above paired case report. I have observed with incredulity the attempts of DSS Medical Officers to squeeze the subjective model of disability into nice tick boxes and scores. Sometimes the attempt is crass or cruel, and it's time for another weary GP letter. Sometimes it's the final way of saying to a patient "OK, your health isn't perfect, but you're not too bad either. You may as well just get on with your life like the rest of us." Is one to be sympathetic, risking collusion, or honest and risk them not knowing how to cope? When the state sponsors disability irrespective of disease it gets to be a complicated business. There is little help to be had from a biomedical model.

Sometimes serendipity demonstrates just how fragile a construct disability really is:

Case report

Mr and Mrs Smith were a devoted couple in their mid-70s. Mrs Smith has been in a wheelchair for many years due to arthritis of the knees and contracted scars on her lower leg due to old complications of surgery following trauma. Mr Smith pushes his wife everywhere in the chair. They seem to function together as a unit, remaining active, with no complaints.

All is well until Mr Smith develops Parkinson's disease. Despite the best efforts of the local Neurologist he gradually becomes immobile. There is a gap of some months when they are seen by my partners. When they next come to see me I am astounded to see Mr Smith in the wheelchair, being pushed into the consulting room by his wife. The situation appeared quite stable, with neither partner complaining. They continued together as a well functioning unit with reversal of their previous roles for a couple of years until Mr Smith died.

Mrs Smith is now in her mid-80s. She remains mobile. She had received no specific medical, surgical or rehabilitative intervention at any point.

I have seen a second case where, in a stable trio of husband, wife and wheelchair the wheelchair user and pusher seamlessly swapped roles with no apparent disruption of their functioning together as a complete unit. As an example of social pathology one could call this "Wheelchair Swapping Syndrome". Mrs Smith made no claim to any particular recovery. Her change in function was implicitly recognised by all concerned simply as a result of her changed circumstances, and the need for her to function according to her social roles, first as a carer and later as a widow.

Disability as escape

Sometimes patients may need to retreat into disability in order to escape from internal pressures. Irritable Bowel Syndrome (IBS) is well recognised as having a large psychological component. Chiotakakou-Faliakou brings a new twist to this particular tale:

Literature review

Chiotakakou-Faliakou E, Dave U and Forbes A, 1996. Wheelchair use: A physical sign in gastroenterological practice. Journal of the Royal Society of Medicine; 89 (9): 490–2.

The authors reviewed 300 consecutive new referrals to a gastroenterology clinic. These included 10 wheelchair users. Four of these used their wheelchairs solely because they found their abdominal symptoms too severe to allow them to walk, without any specific lower limb symptoms. At 1-year follow-up all four had the final diagnosis of "functional symptoms". All four used their wheelchairs regularly.

> The authors comment that "Wheelchair attendance at the gastroenterology clinic, in the absence of lower limb symptoms, is a rare observation, but one that may usefully be added to criteria for diagnosis of a functional disorder."

Escape from normal social responsibilities may include an attempt to escape from ourselves and our own internal problems. Humans are problem solvers. Sometimes sickness is a more achievable solution for internal problems than is change.

The road to sickness

So, apart from those with major physical pathology, who ends up in a sick role? There seems to be a number of factors:

Childhood. Whitehead et al identify childhood modeling as an important determinant of adult sick role behaviour.[8] The way in which parents respond to children's symptoms (reinforcement), and the way parents cope with their own symptoms (modeling) both have a powerful effect in adult life on the number of days off work and the frequency of consultations with a doctor. The number of days off school a child has for URTIs will determine the number of days off work they will have in adult life. (Perhaps this paper should be included in the antenatal pack given to all new parents?)

Social networks. In close communities or social networks "being healthy" is part of what determines one's place within the community.[9] Whether one is seen as healthy may be arrived at by negotiation and consensus between oneself and the group.

Culture. Zola describes ethnic differences in sick role susceptibility.[10] Culture changes with time. Recently a charming 87-year-old said to me "We're still the same as when we were young." They have been married for 68 years and are now very frail with not inconsiderable pathology, but they clearly do not see themselves as sick.

Personality. Alemagno found that "type A" personality patients are more likely than "type B" personality patients to reject the sick role and return to work before they were fully recovered.[11]

Somatisers. Somatisation has been described as "a symptom of a dysfunctional interaction between the patient and their immediate environment, of which the clinician [can become] a significant member".[12] Goldberg argues that somatisation may have three functions:[13]

- It allows people who reject a psychological label, or who live in a culture where mental illness is stigmatised, to occupy the sick role when psychologically unwell.
- It is blame avoiding. Instead of being responsible for problems

arising from one's condition it casts the patient in the role of victim, deserving of help.

• By reducing blame and stigma it may enable a patient to reduce the degree of depression they would otherwise suffer.

Sick role dysfunction

Groves defined four groups of "hateful" patients.[14] These are more commonly called heartsink patients.[15] Grove's four groups are:

The dependant clinger. S/he brings a never-ending stream of symptoms to the doctor, endlessly seeking advice. Whilst grateful for the doctor's efforts s/he is never satisfied, and is dependant on constant reassurance.

The entitled demander. S/he also has an inexhaustible need for health care, but uses demands, intimidation, induction of guilt feelings and threats. The doctor is seen as a barrier to them obtaining their legitimate needs, and is therefore an enemy to be overcome.

The manipulative help rejecter. S/he returns repeatedly to the surgery to complain that the treatment has not worked. Nothing will work! The doctor feels therapeutically impotent, if not therapeutically castrated. And if an intervention does work another problem will appear, and the destructive cycle begins again.

The self destructive denier. S/he is the diabetic in renal failure who won't comply with treatment, and won't stop smoking. The doctor feels as if they are banging their head against a brick wall.

What the four groups have in common is that they're not playing the game. Our view of how the social contract of health care works is to have patients come to us when it is medically necessary, to follow our advice, to get better, and to be grateful to us. This is the social role of the doctor, adjusted to suit the doctor's needs. If the patient doesn't conform to this social role they become our heartsinks.

Labelling

Medical management often works on pattern recognition followed by management by autopilot. If I see an isolated red scaly discoid lesion on the skin, more active and more palpable at the edge, then I reach for an antifungal cream. If I see someone whose spouse has just died then I am aware that they are likely to be grieving, and that this may contain elements such as shock and anger, etc. I don't work out every case I see from basic principles, but I use my past experience to enable me to cut to the chase.

The problem is that sometimes my assumptions will be wrong. Sometimes the ringworm will be discoid eczema. Sometimes the spouse will not be grieving. But if pattern recognition is available it will usually give me the right answer, so it is an efficient tool overall. I can reduce the chance of error if I test out my ideas, particularly looking for any data that doesn't fit.[16]

The social construct of sickness has quite independent roots from biomedical disease, but many of our responses are processed in a similar way. A tubigrip or a wheelchair will label someone as ill or disabled. We may know that they have diagnosis X, therefore we label them as sick. But then the problem starts. We make assumptions on the basis of this sickness label. "They have a tubigrip on their leg: they won't want to play squash this week. They are wheelchair bound with MS: they won't want to come on a winter skiing holiday. They are depressed: they won't want to start a new adult education course." These assumptions may be true, but sometimes they are not.

Labelling is a form of prejudice – a short cut, pre-judging an issue. It gives a standard socially normal response to a given situation. It judges what is needed by seeing the person as a stereotype, drawn from the aggregated files of our subconscious. This doesn't mean it's wrong! It is an example of what Psychologists call "cognitive economy" – it gives us a quick best-bet answer that saves us the trouble of working everything out from scratch. It enables us to arrive at eight right answers and two wrong ones in the time it would otherwise take to generate just one right answer. It is a pragmatic way of dealing with the world. It is dangerous, but it is possible to mitigate against error by testing hypotheses and looking for evidence that doesn't fit.

A classic example of labelling is contained in the title of the BBC Radio 4 programme for the disabled "Does He Take Sugar?". If someone is in a wheelchair we remove some of their social responsibilities (such as changing lightbulbs and digging over the potato bed). This is helpful and appropriate. But it is also automatic, and not specific to their exact situation. So all sorts of inappropriate responses get pulled in too – we ask their companion "does he take sugar?". Wheelchair and all, they can still decide for themselves whether to take sugar, go on a skiing trip or start a new job.

Much of a patient's experience of illness actually depends on the reactions of those around them. Society tends to label different illnesses in different ways.[17] Many of these labelling effects help patients. Some just seem designed to drive them wild.

Labellers – what, us?

I have described labelling as a part of society's response to the patient. But doctors label their patients too. Blalock and Devellis found that doctors bend their use of information depending on their stereotypical models of the "type" of patients they are treating.[18] Armitage found that physicians tend to take the same symptoms more seriously in men than in women.[19] Jeffery found that casualty officers sort people into "good" and "bad" patients, the good being deserving of care, and the bad being labelled as "normal rubbish".[20]

Labelling patients helps us to cope with treating them in bulk – a task that the NHS demands of us. But we do this at the expense of reaching a deeper understanding of our patients as individuals, and this impoverishes the help that we can offer them.

This was brought home to me powerfully when I had been in my current practice about a year:

Case report [with personal notes]

Before I went to Medical School I respected my elders. Putting so many of them into pyjamas in hospital wards where they became passive recipients of my expertise seemed to damage that. I suppose like many young people the elderly were a bit of a remote group for me. I wanted to show understanding and care, because they often had the greatest medical needs, and had to cope with the greatest disabilities, but I expect I always found it hard to see them as real people. They didn't seem to function the same way as me.

Ivy was in her 70s, and suffered from extensive osteoarthritis and heart failure. Her mobility was poor, and she used two sticks. I couldn't cure her. She was yet another old lady who I would have to do my best to help, with damage limitation, Occupational Therapy assessment, analgesics and of course my wise and encouraging words.

I can't even remember why I asked about her past level of activity. She told me about her youth. She had excelled at athletics at school, and was encouraged to compete for her county. She trained hard and continued to win, until she reached the pinnacle of her achievement, being picked for the British Squad in the 1936 Berlin Olympic Games.

I was astounded. As a child my father had told me about the 1936 Olympics, when Hitler had been determined to prove the superiority of his "master race". The black American athlete Jesse Owens had frustrated the Nazis' efforts by winning four gold medals. These games were played out against the backdrop of the rise of Fascism and the mounting danger of the 1930s. The whole event had been a dramatic prelude to the war.

My father's account had captured my imagination. Those games had become a legend. And now part of that legend was here in my consulting room. This frail old lady in front of me was one of those who had struggled to deny Hitler the victories he craved.

So was she a frail old lady, or was she a hero? I suddenly understood that she was both. That old people are people like me too. That many of Ivy's generation had memories of courage and achievement that I could never guess.

What Ivy taught me has helped me to look after many other hidden heroes. I have tried to learn the roads my older patients have travelled. The anxious old lady with the troublesome glass eye becomes the stoical survivor of the Blitz, buried under the rubble of her house for two days, with only the corpses of her family for company. The senior citizen who always appears agitated and hypochondriacal becomes the damaged victim of a Japanese concentration camp. The uninteresting old man with constipation becomes the soldier driving his tank up the beach on D-Day.

Labelling is OK so long as we constantly test and challenge it. Labelling is not OK if we use it as a means to hide from the people who come to us with real needs from their real and unique lives.

Stigma

The sick role has another murky corner. Stigma is an example of inappropriate labelling. Many diseases carry a stigma. Obvious examples would be epilepsy, facial disfigurement, mental illness and HIV. Stigma therefore becomes an additional complication of that individual's sick role.

Stigma relies on attaching a significance on a particular feature, and using it to define the "one of us/not one of us" boundary. Stigma only exists within a social context – it is socially constructed. Stigma takes a personal feature, such as a diagnostic label, and attaches a social meaning. Waxler showed that, in the case of leprosy, patients learn that various ways of relating and living are closed off to them, not because of the disease process itself but because of the social significance attached to the diagnosis.[21] Stigma is therefore tribalism against one individual in a group:

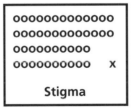

Scambler showed that stigma is a game that takes two to play.[22] Some groups have been successful in rejecting the offer of stigmatisation, e.g. being gay could have been said to carry a stigma 20 years ago, but this is less so now. Similarly people with mental illness, through organisations such as MIND, are seeking to challenge and gradually dump their own burden of stigma.

Stigma tends to produce shame in individuals and fear in others. This adds to the burden of illness that the patient already suffers. Stigma is a form of prejudice which doctors should be ready to challenge.

Responsibility – free will or an oppressive social construct?

Jane Ogden, a tutor on the Guys, Kings and St Thomas' MSc in General Practice, said "We want people to take responsibility for their health, but we don't want to blame them when they get sick."[23] Responsibility is a tricky concept.

Responsibility is rarely black and white. How do we construct a concept of responsibility if we are told Mr Black, a smoker for 40 years, has lung cancer?

> **Option 1:** Mr Black is responsible for becoming ill because he smokes.
> **Option 2:** Mr Black is not responsible for his illness, because he was targeted with advertising for an addictive drug whilst he was young, subject to peer pressure, and in no position to come to an adult choice.

Which option is correct? I guess it depends on which way you vote.

Ninety-three per cent of people in a poll agreed with the statement: "If I take the right actions, I can stay healthy."[24] Brownell points out that the idea of empowerment may have negative consequences.[25] Do we really believe, with the 93% of those polled, that our health lies mainly in our own hands? Holding an individual responsible for a misfortune that is not under their control is called "victim blaming". Victim blaming is the downside of strong models of personal responsibility.

In reality there is a continuous spectrum. How would you rate the degree of personal responsibility in the following situations?

	Individual is	
	responsible	*not responsible*
Loses a week's earnings on the horses	|_|_|_|_|_|_|_|_|_|_|	
Loses a month's salary on stockmarket	|_|_|_|_|_|_|_|_|_|_|	
Loses a month's salary on stockmarket through taking financial adviser's advice	|_|_|_|_|_|_|_|_|_|	
Develops Huntingdon's Chorea	|_|_|_|_|_|_|_|_|_|	
OA knee worsens, overweight	|_|_|_|_|_|_|_|_|_|	
OA knee worsens, not overweight	|_|_|_|_|_|_|_|_|_|	
OA knee worsens, rugby player	|_|_|_|_|_|_|_|_|_|	
OA knee worsens, carpet layer	|_|_|_|_|_|_|_|_|_|	

Unless you decided this exercise was meaningless and that you wouldn't play I hope this has demonstrated that you have some criteria in your mind which:

1 determine whether someone carries some degree of responsibility for outcome or not;

2 determine the relative force of different factors in establishing the degree of responsibility.

So how can you validate your views on point 2, other than by admitting they are part of your own pet social model?

Perhaps both freedom and responsibility are rather like the location of an electron. It is not possible to say where it is located at any given moment, but the further away from the "expected" place you look the less is its probability of being there. We are all free within limits. But the further we stray from the social norm the harder it is to exercise that freedom.

Similarly we may be held responsible for our actions. But our actions are not the result of our own volition, operating within a vacuum. Our volition operates within a recipe that includes social forces from without and cognitive systems from within.

Conclusions

Norms for illness behaviour are socially defined. If the patient believes they are ill then a pattern of behaviours called the sick role will tend to occur. For the sick role to be legitimised socially it must be recognised by a doctor. The sick role relieves patients of responsibility. Thus, like any winning move, it is liable to be bent and misused, and to end up surrounded with confusing rules. Both doctors and patients are affected by the ambivalence and dysfunction inevitable in the grinding crash between medical pathology and socially constructed sickness.

References

1 Zola I, 1973. Pathways to the doctor – from person to patient. Social Science and Medicine; 7: 677–89.

2 Zola I, 1973. Pathways to the doctor – from person to patient. Social Science and Medicine; 7: 677–89.

3 Friedson E, 1960. Client control and medical practice. American Journal of Sociology; 65: 374–82.

4 Cornford C and Cornford H, 1999. "I'm only here because of my family." A study of lay referral networks. British Journal of General Practice; 49: 617–20.

5 Ajzen I and Madden T, 1986. Prediction of goal-directed behaviour: Attitudes, intentions and perceived behavioural control. Journal of experimental Social Psychology; 22: 453–74.

6 Parsons T, 1951. The social system. New York: Free Press.

7 Armstrong D, 1989. An outline of sociology as applied to medicine. 3rd edition. London: Wright. Chapter 2, p. 7.

8 Whitehead W et al, 1994. Modeling and reinforcement of the sick role during childhood predicts adult illness behaviour. Psychosomatic Medicine; 56 (6): 541–50.

9 Litva A and Eyles J 1994. Health or healthy: Why people are not sick in a southern Ontarian town. Social Science and Medicine; 39: 1083–91.

10 Zola I, 1973. Pathways to the doctor – from person to patient. Social Science and Medicine; 7: 677–89.

11 Alemagno S et al, 1991. Health and illness behaviour of type A persons. Journal of Occupational Medicine; 33: 891–5.

12 Vandereycken W and Meermann R, 1988. Chronic illness behaviour and noncompliance with treatment: pathways to an interactive approach. Psychotherapy and Psychosomatics; 50: 182–91.

13 Goldberg D and Bridges K, 1988. Somatic presentations of psychiatric illness in primary care setting. Journal of Psychosomatic Research; 32: 137–44.

14 Groves J, 1951. Taking care of the hateful patient. New England Journal of Medicine; 298: 883–5.

15 O'Dowd T, 1988. Five years of heartsink patients in general practice. BMJ; 297: 528–30.

16 Sackett D et al, 1991. Clinical epidemiology, a basic science for clinical medicine. 2nd edn. Boston: Little, Brown and Co. Chap 1.

17 Freidson E, 1970. Profession of medicine. New York: Aldine. Chap 11.

18 Blalock S and Devellis B, 1986. Stereotyping: the link between theory and practice. Patient Education and Counselling; 8: 17–25.

19 Armitage K et al, 1979. Response of physicians to medical complaints in men and women. JAMA; 241: 2186–7.

20 Jeffery R, 1979. Normal rubbish: deviant patients in casualty departments. Sociology of Health and Illness; 1: 90–107.

21 Waxler N, 1981. Learning to be a leper: a case study in the social construction of illness. In Mishler et al (eds), Social context of health, illness and patient care. Cambridge: Cambridge University Press.

22 Scambler G and Hopkins A, 1986. Being epileptic: coming to terms with stigma. Sociology of Health and Illness; 8: 26–43.

23 Ogden J, 1996. Personal communication.

24 Glassner B, 1988. Bodies: Why we look the way we do and how we feel about it. New York: Putnam.

25 Brownell K, 1991. Personal responsibility and control over our bodies: When expectation exceeds reality. Health Psychology; 10: 303–10.

7 Sociological models:
ii Medicalisation

The medical establishment has become a major threat to health.

Ivan Illich, the opening sentence of *Medical Nemesis*[1]

The roads to unfreedom are many. Signposts on one of them bear the inscription HEALTH FOR ALL.

Petr Skrabanek, the opening sentence of *The Death of Humane Medicine*[2]

A well person is a patient who has not been completely worked up.

Freymann[3]

Chapter summary

Illness behaviour is culturally determined. A sociological model of illness exposes problems in our biomedical healthcare model. These problems have a negative effect on both individual patients and society as a whole.

Making illness

The WHO defines health as "not merely the absence of disease or infirmity but a state of complete physical, mental and social well-being". But this Utopian vision is an unattainable ideal, bearing no relation to the struggles of real people in an imperfect world. The WHO definition however represents the aim of the biomedical model. If we are closed, knowable systems then imperfections should be fixed. Logically, as none of us is in this complete state of wellbeing, we are all in need of medical intervention to correct whatever "abnormalities" obstruct our path to perfection. But should we view any deviation from perfection as pathology needing treatment? Where do we draw the line?

As I write this book I glance up from time to time to look at our garden. It's not just a technique for avoiding eye strain, I love our garden. But the garden isn't perfect. It has inherent conflicts of purpose – it has to satisfy both football-crazed children and tranquillity-seeking adults. It will never get into a TV show. It is green and peaceful but a bit unfinished and wild around the edges. My garden is important to me, but in reality I balance the time and money I spend on it against the other priorities in my life, and I don't expect it to be perfect.

Imagine however if when I went to a garden centre I was met by an authoritative figure who, when I asked if they had an evergreen fermontodendron, first insisted on inspecting my garden, and then followed this up with a list of detailed reccommendations of the work that I should be putting into my garden week by week.

OK, gardens and health care aren't the same. Yes, there is more at stake (I can always get another garden). But the issue of whether I think it worthwhile to let an expert take control of my life is the same. The personal issue of weighing up my own priorities is the same. Don't we tend to take over our patients' health agenda rather too easily? Don't we tend to assume that health-related issues should be dealt with according to medical rules rather than the patient's rules?

The retreat of the well

Medicine exists to reduce the burden of disease. The problem with targeting every minor deviance from normality for treatment is that this actually increases the number of "medical problems" out there without reducing disease by the same amount. The more we classify minor abnormality as disease then the less well people we will have:

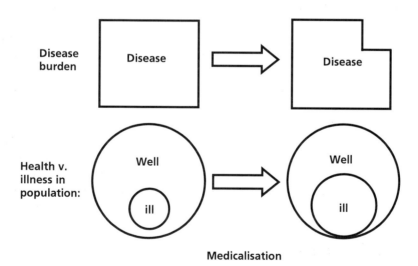

Medicalisation

Clifton Meador, in a satirical article in the *New England Journal of Medicine*, pictures the discovery of the last well person.[4] Meador comments "If the behaviour of doctors and the public continues unabated, eventually every well person will be labeled sick... We will all be assigned to one diagnosis-related group or another... Who will be the last well person? How will that person avoid diagnostic labels?" Meador pictures a man who devotes 7 hours a day to the task of staying healthy, who has repeated screening tests to check on his health, and whose lifestyle is dominated by his health beliefs. Fit perhaps, but fit for what?

If I enquire about a new car and find my personal cost–benefit equation doesn't work out then I walk away. I'm then sent a series of reminders and offers in the post. We call it junk mail, which is bad. If my doctor finds I have an asymptomatic risk factor such as a mildly raised blood pressure or cholesterol I might also weigh up the personal cost–benefit equation and, perhaps after trying the advice for a while, decide to walk away. I then get a series of reminders in the post. But this time we call it medical follow-up, which is good. I am labelled a "non-complier", which smacks of social deviance tantamount to a moral lapse. Should we not instead see adequately informed non-compliance as a reasonable adult choice?

Medicalisation of life problems

Medicalisation leads to a pathological society, with less good health and more sick people.

Consider the difficulty in the diagnosis of depression. The "Defeat Depression" campaign of the Royal College of Psychiatrists and Royal College of General Practitioners urges doctors to "increase … the recognition and effective treatment of depression".[5] But there is a slight problem. What is "depression"? It's more difficult to define than a broken leg. Depression is a medical construct, recognising a number of different features, and postulating a link through a biomedical pathology. Depression would not be recognised in the same way in other cultures, or here in the West in other centuries. Furthermore it is unclear whether making a definitive diagnosis of depression reliably improves the outcome for the patient.[6]

But the Psychiatrists have it all sorted out. You're depressed if you score beyond a certain threshold of a formal Psychiatric rating scale.[7,8] This emphasises the nature of depression as a medical construct. Such scales may be very helpful when dealing with a selected subgroup of the population referred to Psychiatrists by GPs. Problems arise when one tries to implement "rating scale" diagnosis in the general population, as Kessler et al found out:

Literature review

Kessler D, Lloyd L, Lewis G, and Pereira Gray D, 1999. Cross sectional study of symptom attribution and recognition of depression and anxiety in primary care. BMJ; 318: 436–40.

This study administered a general health questionnaire to 355 consecutive adult patients attending one GP surgery. 305 patients completed questionnaires.

52% of the responders had GHQ scores categorising them as suffering from pathological anxiety or depression. GPs diagnosed pathological anxiety or depression in 24% of patients. GPs were less likely to make a psychological diagnosis in patients with a high GHQ score where patients explained their symptoms with reference to other causes, such as physical illness. The authors conclude patients' tendency to explain their low feelings by reference to other factors (especially physical factors) is "an important cause of low detection rates [by GPs] of depression and anxiety".

Iona Heath, in a commentary on this study, notes that a "staggering 51.5% of the patients were considered by the researchers to have measurable depression. This extraordinary finding does not seem to have disturbed them."[9] Are these people really depressed in any meaningful medical sense, or are the GHQ scores simply reflective of the distress of being ill or stressed enough to want to see a doctor? Is this paper an example of inappropriate medicalisation of "normal" human distress?

What about screening?

How much of our lives do we want to spend on guarding against medical risk? In the USA Frame and Carlson recommend that a perfectly healthy woman seeking no special advice should, between the ages of 40 and 65, have 13 BP checks, 1 cholesterol check, 6 smears, 14 breast examinations, 14 checks of breast self-examination technique, 11 mammograms, 13 stool occult bloods, 3 tetanus immunisations, 6 smoking history checks, 6 alcohol history checks, 6 family function enquiries, 1 session of menopause counselling and one session of pre-retirement counselling. McWhinney in Canada advocates routine screening of healthy adults at specified intervals for hypertension, cholesterol, cancer of colon, cancer of rectum, oral cancer, skin cancer, alcohol problems, smoking, family dysfunction, marital and sexual problems, hearing impairment, retirement problems, and additional checks for women for hypothyroidism, smears, breast cancer and osteoporosis.[10]

But surely it's all harmless fun and only good can result? Let us look at hypertension screening. Hart states: "It is now generally accepted that management of uncomplicated high blood pressure implies continuing care of some sort (with or without medication) for between 10 and 30% of the adult population."[11] Hart also cites evidence that "at least one third of American 60 year olds with access to medical care are currently treated with antihypertensive drugs." And this for a condition with an NNT of 850 per year? What about side effects?

So what is the evidence?

In 1978 Haynes showed that labelling a patient hypertensive led to an 80% increase in absenteeism from work, regardless of whether treatment was given.[12] Awareness that they had an "unhealthy" blood pressure made these patients feel themselves to be unhealthy, and they therefore became unhealthy.

More alarmingly still Jachuck et al found that relatives noticed adverse effects in patients diagnosed as hypertensive.[13] These included preoccupation with sickness, decline in energy, decline in general activity, decline in sexual activity and irritability. These effects were measured by the Quality of Life Impairment Scale (QLIS), and were classed as severe in 30% of patients.

As a pilot to a small research study I tried a little exercise. I asked 10 consecutive hypertensive patients three questions:

- Do you ever wonder if you might be getting side effects from your medication?
- Do you often think about your blood pressure?
- Does your blood pressure cause you any problems in your day-to-day life?

Remember that these were healthy patients in whom I was seeking to modify a risk factor, not treat a disease. And this risk factor will never harm most of them anyway. I was alarmed to find eight negative effects in five of the ten patients:

- Two descriptions of mild ("acceptable") side effects – morning dieuresis.
- For three patients, their asymptomatic hypertension provided a frequent source of anxious thoughts ("Yes, I worry every day". "I try not to think [about it], but then I think 'Oh crikey, stroke!' " "I wonder what effect it will have when I get other illnesses.")
- Three patients described evidence that it stigmatised, or had the potential to stigmatise, them with family or friends. ("My family protects me … there is a list of 'mustn't does'." "My friends tell me horror stories [about the risks of 'blood pressure']." "I've not told my family that I have blood pressure [because I would find it difficult to do so]." For one patient there was a "positive stigma" – two work colleagues were hypertensive; they discussed their treatment together and it clearly formed a positive and supportive bond between them.

Why not try this exercise yourself?

If labelling a patient as "sick" for a supposedly asymptomatic risk factor can actually make a patient sick then what about the intervention of screening itself?

Screening programmes for cervical cancer, breast cancer and general health screens can generate high levels of anxiety.[14,15] This may constitute a significant disbenefit to patients, as anxiety is unpleasant, can cause illness itself, and can reduce patients' ability to cope and to recall relevant health information.[16]

But are there any negative effects from screening beyond anxiety?

Literature Review

Stoate H, 1989. Can health screening damage your health? Journal of the Royal College of General Practitioners; 39: 193–5.

Stoate administered the Goldberg general health questionnaire before and three months after screening examinations on a group of 215 patients aged 35–65 years in whom no abnormalities were found. These were compared with a matched group of 225 unscreened controls. This questionnaire measures psychological distress, and has been found to correlate with perceived health status. There were two significant findings.

First the GHQ scores of those attending for screening were significantly better than the control group. This suggests that Hart's inverse care law is operating – those with a better health status are the ones who attend for screening.[17]

The second finding was novel. Whilst there was no significant change in the two GHQ scores three months apart in the control group, the GHQ scores in the screening group were significantly worse three months after the screening examination. The meaning of the reduction in wellbeing is far from clear. None the less the finding that screening leads to a significant increase in psychological distress (or decreased perception of health status) at three months is alarming.

Stoate speculates that "this type of systematic screening may have made some people more aware of their mortality and more hypochondriacal, leading to greater psychological distress. If patients become more dependent on health services to deal with their life problems this has serious implications, not only for patients themselves but for the health services."

We must question whether medical pursuit of all undesirable biomedical indices promotes health. Will our grandchildren decide that it makes about as much sense as bloodletting? We all surely must have risk factors for something. The screening model suggested by Wilson works well if, without any harm to the "normal" majority, we are able to identify a subgroup who will clearly benefit from risk free intervention.[18] We must therefore ask certain questions:

- Is screening harmless? Surely the evidence that it creates anxiety, increased perception of vulnerability and behavioural changes suggests that it is not.
- Does the personal probability of benefit justify the risk of iatrogenic illness, such as side effects or complications from interventions?
- Are we confusing statistical significance with clinical significance? Although an intervention may achieve statistically significant benefit for a population, if an individual's personal probability of benefit is actually low is it helpful to intervene in their lives given that intervention may be harmful? Davey Smith showed that, as the benefit

of an intervention may apply to only a few of those treated but the disbenefits apply to the whole treatment group, then the significance of this effect is magnified.[19]

Surveillance medicine

Armstrong argues that "a new medicine based on the surveillance of normal populations can be identified as emerging in the twentieth century. This new surveillance medicine involves a fundamental remapping of the spaces of illness. This includes the problematisation of normality, the redrawing of the relationship between symptom, sign and illness, and the localisation of illness outside the corporal space of the body."[20]

Armstrong takes our previous classification of bedside medicine and hospital medicine one step further:

Step 1: Bedside medicine (17th century)
The symptom is the illness to be treated. Ill people need medical care.
Step 2: Hospital and laboratory medicine (18th–mid-20th century)
The symptom indicates there is a hidden disease. This must be located within the body and treated. Diseases require medical intervention.
Step 3: Surveillance medicine (late 20th century)
No symptoms, but illness is not restricted to being unwell. Illness is not only a physical problem located in the body, but a concept of devience from normality which requires treatment. Everyone needs medical care.

Foucault points out that the reference point of bedside medicine is "health", whereas the reference point of hospital medicine is "normality".[21] It's not enough to say you're well. Surveillance medicine reaches the parts of the population other medical interventions cannot reach.

Preventionitis

The enthusiastic belief that prevention must be better than cure has been labelled "preventionitis". Perhaps the most vigorous critic of this belief was Petr Skrabanek:

Book review

The Death of Humane Medicine. Petr Skrabanek. The Social Affairs Unit, London, 1994.

Skrabanek was an Associate Professor in the Department of Community Health in Trinity College Dublin, having left Czechoslovakia in 1968. The theme of the book is revealed in its subtitle, "The rise of coercive healthism". The book starts with the statement quoted at the beginning of the chapter: "The roads to unfreedom are many. Signposts on one of them bear the inscription HEALTH FOR ALL."

The book propounds three ideas:

- First, Skrabanek describes the pursuit of health as a state ideology as "healthism". He observes that there has been a change from "old style doctoring, which was in the main the care of the sick, to a new style of 'anticipatory' care". It is no longer enough to be free of sickness. We should all be attempting to approach the WHO definition's state of perfection, as penitents seeking absolution. "Health" has thereby become an unattainable yet commercialised product, promoted by healthcare managers, and driven by the state.

- Second, he describes unrealistic attempts to avoid illness and death by lifestyle changes as "lifestylism". He does not mean by this a lifestyle change that has a clear benefit for an individual (such as a bronchitic stopping smoking or an obese arthritic losing weight). He refers to an overvalued belief in lifestyle changes, to be urged upon whole populations. He criticises many lifestyle recommendations as being driven more by social or political fashion than by evidence. We cope with death and disease by denial, and use lifestylism as a form of magical thinking, seeking to avert them.

- Third, he coins the term "coercive medicine" to describe what he sees as the medical profession's attempts to gain power over peoples' lives, in collusion with the growth of the state, and influenced by financial incentives. Health education backed by political force and divorced from evidence becomes propaganda. Doctors act as agents of the state. The medical profession has fallen prey to a desire to control others, supplanting our traditional responsibility to care for the sick.

Skrabanek's book is a grand polemic. It argues that the Health Promotion Emperor has no clothes. It supplies referenced evidence, and a socio-political background for its arguments. It forces us to reflect on the role of our profession in society, and upon our own motives as doctors.

I guess this is not a black and white issue. I'm not saying we should never take a blood pressure or check a baby's hips. But we should look more critically at the evidence for benefit from surveillance medicine in terms of actual outcomes (not intermediate outcomes). This then needs to be balanced against the evidence for harm from surveillance intervention. And we need as much research into harm from intervention as there is for benefit. (And we must consider that even this is a very doctor-centred view. Where is the view of our major stakeholder, the patient?)

We need to locate this issue within the context of our beliefs about a healthy society. To quote Armstrong again, do we really want the "new public health dream of surveillance in which everyone is brought into the vision of the benevolent eye of medicine through the medicalisation of everyday life"?[22] If the 20th century has taught us anything, surely it is that we should not surrender to any narrow dogma that promises perfection. Popper has reminded us to be suspicious of grand visions and final solutions.[23] The world is a profoundly imperfect place, and our attempts to better it should be founded on concrete evidence of benefit, not on Utopian fantasy.

The dark side of medicine?

Are Armstrong and Skrabanek right? If so, why is medicine like this? There is no single answer to these questions. What answers we may find depend on looking at how our medical system works.

George Bernard Shaw said, "all professions are conspiracies against the laity".[24] We are part of a profession that exists for the benefit of patients. But we also have needs ourselves. How much is the profession of medicine structured for the benefit of patients, and how much is it structured for our own benefit? Is it sometimes true, as Wilmshurst asserts, that "clinical performance and welfare of patients often come second to the interests of institutions and loyalty to colleagues"?[25]

Freidson argues that doctors dominate patients.[26] He sees doctors as maintaining professional dominance by controlling an exclusive license to practice medicine, prescribe drugs, refer to specialists and admit patients. We hold a powerful monopoly.[27] Beyond these specific rights held exclusively by doctors is the broader cultural authority of medicine.[28] We normally hold the balance of power in our consulting rooms. Our ethics call on us to use that power for the good of patients, but we can hardly maintain that we never use any of it for our own comfort too.

If you're getting twitchy at this point I would express my own view that none of this is wrong in itself. A rabidly pro-patient activist may demand that I see every patient when and where they want for as long as they want and give them every test and treatment that they want. But if these changes were implemented patients would find that some of these rights were mutually incompatible, and they would be serviced by a rapidly diminishing body of burnt-out doctors. Any social system has to maintain a balance of interests. The question is not "Do we hold monopoly powers?" – we do. The question is "Have we got the balance of interests right?" If we cannot address this question effectively ourselves then the government will be only to happy to address it for us.

Ivan Illich did the medical profession a great service by launching a blistering attack upon us in the 1970s.[29] He makes three accusations:

1 Doctors are useless. Their attempt to reduce society's burden of illness doesn't work.
2 Doctors have organised medicine for their own good, contrary to the interests of patients.
3 Doctors exert inappropriate social control by turning normal human problems into medical problems ("medical imperialism").

My personal answer to Illich's first accusation was contained in Chapter 1. I would say we are of use. Perhaps not as much as our preferred Dr Kildare image would imply, but we're still the best show in town, and it matters.

Illich does us a favour in his other two accusations. Without the proper action of osteoclasts bones become Pagetic. Without the action of iconoclasts social institutions become overgrown and dysfunctional. Illich forces us to consider the dark side of medicine.

Medical imperialism?

Medicine is an expansionist project. We even hold "outreach clinics". Medicine seeks to expand into the greenfield sites of human existance with its command and control solutions to problems no-one knew they had.

It would be a mistake to see doctors as the only driving force behind medicalisation. There are five main driving forces behind medicine's expansion.

Doctors

I have described Armstrong's concept of the medicalisation of normality on page 139. Yesterday's fit and healthy elder is today's hypertensive patient, processed, medicated and monitered.

Patients

Patients can play the medicalisation game well enough themselves. It is debatable whether we taught them or whether the game is innate (see Chapter 8). I guess it's a bit of both. But who can blame patients for a "buy loads, come again" philosophy if we make big claims. Instead of taking responsibility for problems with the support of friends we seek counselling. We seek antibiotics for self-limiting complaints. We seek a somatic diagnosis to camouflage distress. We seek a prescription or a certificate to shield us from the perils of daily life.

Holloway describes a syndrome of over-compliance with medical advice which, in Latin America, is termed susto.[30] Patients who pick up on every suggestion and implication of medical advice can end up more disabled than those who simply get on with life as best they can. Doctors' tendency to be cautious and keep a margin of safety therefore works against the patient's best interest.

I remember a 51-year-old lady who came to see me requesting exemption from jury service on the grounds of her asthma. I was rather surprised as her asthma was extremely mild. The discussion became rather dysfunctional until I finally realised that her concern was that she was illiterate, a fact she generally concealed, and she was concerned that she would be humiliated. Her preferred solution was to medicalise her dilemma.

Society

In 1766 the Empress Maria Theresa decided that the court physicians should certify prisoners as fit for torture.[31] Ever since then we have been expected to be the arbiters of a multitude of social, rather than medical, decisions which bear no relation to any therapeutic process.

The request for a certificate to confirm that a patient had gained weight so that she could claim for new clothes from Social Services has little to do with medicine. Seeking to define who is "vulnerable" and eligible for emergency housing by use of a biomedical model is similarly problematic.

Politicians

Health care is one of the issues that decide general election results. We are the victims of our own success. Politicians naturally want a Rolls Royce healthcare service for the cost of a Skoda. There is therefore increasing pressure to apply a biomedical model as efficiently as possible. That's great where a biomedical model is appropriate, but a side effect is the extension of medical guidelines into an ever greater part of the nation's life.

A hot area in this debate is the role of psychiatrists as protectors of the public. Even before the 19th-century Mental Health Act it was accepted that doctors should protect society from the tiny proportion of the mentally ill who pose a threat to others. Not content with this, politicians now want doctors to protect society not just from the "mad" but from the "bad" also, by extending their role in detaining those with personality disorder. Eastman comments: "The fragility of the distinction between public health psychiatry and crime prevention has never before been so starkly represented as it is now in this proposal. However all doctors should note the subtle but growing social requirement that medical practice should be applied towards public protection. That requirement is not restricted to the practice of forensic psychiatry".[32]

Commerce

"Are you getting cross for no reason? Are colleagues getting it in the neck? Are you taking it out on the ones you love most? ... A bed that is ten years old or more may not be giving you the comfort and support you need for a good healthy night's sleep ... So if you buy a new bed, you could soon snap out of it..."[33] This is the actual text from a magazine advert.

The medical model can be used to entice the vulnerable into purchasing not only beds, but also vitamins, tonics, food supplements, gadgets, and dubious therapies of every kind.

Medicine as social control

This is a game that any can play. Here are a couple of real requests that have been made to me. I relay them as they are, completely unembellished:

> **Note (left at reception by patient's wife)**
>
> Further to Saturday the heating is still broken and the council can't come until tomorrow. Mrs X said you needed to know.

If the problem was hypothermia, fair enough. For an active middle-aged man with stable angina in a Western society which has ready access to electric heaters, is the use of a medical model appropriate?

> **Telephone message (as written in message book)**
>
> Mrs Y phoned. Requests a letter for the council to say that her 2 daughters A and B suffer from asthma and would benefit from the installation of a bath. (They have a shower at present.)

What we lose

Medicine exists to lessen the burden of disease. When we let it muscle in on other areas of life we lose something. Not all of life's problems are due to disease. Medicalisation of non-medical problems reduces our ability to solve those problems. Let's consider a few examples:

> **Case report**
>
> Mary is a 33-year-old school cook. She was sent to see me by her boss after she had collapsed at work. A clear biomedical problem.
>
> On talking to Mary a different picture emerged. The school's catering budget had been cut, and she was now doing the work previously done by three people. Before her collapse she had been particularly rushed and hassled, and had been working without a rest break. She had been standing for some time preparing food in a hot steamy environment. The collapse itself sounded like a typical vasovagal faint. On examination there were no abnormal findings.
>
> This was the last straw for Mary. She was stressed and weepy, but anxious not to lose her job. I gave her a medical certificate for 10 days, stating "work related stress reaction" as the diagnosis, and discussed with her how she should complain about her working conditions to her boss. She saw no realistic chance of change.

The problem is unreasonable work conditions. The solution is to see the doctor. I'm scarcely a left-wing radical, but I would rather she saw a union representative. But then of course the majority of employees, especially the low-paid, do not have a union representative. I would like to put "unreasonable working conditions" on her certificate, but that is scarcely a medical diagnosis. By medicalising Mary's problem we are depriving her of an acknowledgement that the problem is her working conditions. Whilst her boss is able to label Mary's problem as medical we are lessening the chance of change. And we are lessening her ability to press for change.

I was driving from a conference, listening to a BBC Radio 4 feature on behavioural problems in schools. The feature described the case of a boy who as a result of dysfunctional life experiences was disrupting classes and causing problems to the teacher and other pupils.[34] The reporter continued with a phrase that struck me so forcefully that I had to pull into a lay-by to write it down. Referring to the pupil he stated "He has since been diagnosed with emotional behavioural difficulties". To which we are supposed to reply "Aha, so that explains it." The term "emotional behavioural difficulties" is a description of a human problem, but it is being used as a medical diagnosis. It is not a medical condition. It is not like saying that the child has Tourette's syndrome or autism. It is the equivalent of the patient who sees a dermatologist saying "Doctor, my skin is red", to be told "Aha, that's because you have erythema". A medical condition needs medical treatment, but is a medical model the best way of dealing with a disruptive pupil from a dysfunctional background?

Case report

Jenny is a 37-year-old office manager in a small firm. She usually works a 12-hour day. She found herself lumbered with organising a trip abroad for a charitable social group after the unexpected death of a friend. She is feeling extremely stressed and has become anxious about her ability to cope with her new responsibilities.

She is visibly shaking. Her words to me are "I need tranquillisers".

The problem is this patient's struggle to manage her time and her personal resources, due to her inability to set boundaries. Her perceived solution is pills. I felt this was particularly sad as she was able and articulate, but I guess neither quality guarantees appropriate survival skills. My worry was that the pursuit of tranquillisers, just like a resort to alcohol, reduces her self-reliance and her hardiness, and therefore reinforces her problems rather than improving her ability to solve them.

Letter from Consultant Child Psychiatrist

The letter was drawn from the old records of a single mother who presented with her own parenting difficulties.

"As you know this little girl has been attending this Hospital since **** when she was seen by Dr M … Both parents were full of complaints about X [the patient], about her restlessness and destructiveness. Both parents find X's behaviour intolerable and they feel that they cannot cope with her any longer. They demanded that she should be admitted for treatment or that she should be sent away. None of this behaviour has been observed at school where her behaviour does not constitute a problem…"

Determinedly pushing on the wrong button prevents one from pushing on the right button. So long as these parents see the Psychiatrist as responsible for solving their problem with their daughter they will never take responsibility for solving it themselves. The loser is the daughter, who is now struggling with her attempt not to pass the same lousy deal on to her own children.

We weave reality with words

In all of these examples words are the tools used to medicalise life problems. Words are not used to understand a given reality but rather to create a new reality. This was brought home to me as a young GP when a certificate I had given to a woman whose spouse had tragically been killed in an accident was rejected by the local Department of Social Security office. I had written on the certificate "bereavement". But, doctor, bereavement is a life problem, not a medical diagnosis. With the advice of a wiser colleague I returned the certificate stating "bereavement reaction", and presto, problem solved, medical diagnosis accepted.

The medicalisation of death

Medicine has not yet succeeded in reducing the 100% mortality rate of each generation. Part of our job is to save lives, but we know there are many that cannot be saved. Surely in inevitable deaths best practice in palliative care should be the norm?

We know that many more patients wish to die at home than manage to do so. We attack pathology even when we should be negotiating the terms of surrender. Elizabeth Kubler-Ross said of the dying patient: "He will be surrounded by nurses, orderlies, interns, residents, lab technicians perhaps who will take some blood and an electrocardiogram. He will be moved to X-ray and he will hear and overhear opinions about his condition, discussions and questions to members of his family. He slowly but surely is beginning to be treated like a thing; he is no longer a person".[35]

This was Simone de Beauvoir's experience, in her account of the death of her mother:[36]

A very easy death

I was stepping into another story: instead of a convalescence, a death bed. The scene had changed. The sweets had been put away in cupboards; so had the books. There were no flowers any more on the big table, but bottles, balloon flasks, test tubes. Maman was asleep ... under the bed one could see jars and pipes that connected with her stomach and intestines. Her left arm was attached to an intravenous drip. She was no longer wearing any clothes whatsoever: the bed jacket was spread over her chest and her naked shoulders...

She said, "I hurt all over." She moved her swollen fingers anxiously. Her confidence waned: "These doctors are beginning to irritate me. They are always telling me that I am getting better. And I feel myself getting worse..."

Conclusion

For two hundred years most people in the West have seen autonomy as a desirable. To quote John Stuart Mill: "Over himself, over his own body and mind, the individual is sovereign."[37] We know that the ability to increase control of one's world improves health.[38]

But doctors tend to take control. To a certain extent this is necessary, e.g. in an emergency situation, or in controlling exposure to complex hazards. But even in a non-urgent situation we control. "Take this pill." "Go for this test." "See me in three months." After all, we are the masters of the biomedical model, we know what needs to be done and we've only got ten minutes to do it in. But the more we control them, the less the patients control themselves. That damages the patient's ability to continue to control themselves, which is morally undesirable, and may actually damage their health.

We are keen to avoid dishing out antibiotics without good cause because we now acknowledge the problems this causes. Shouldn't we attempt to limit our control tendencies in the same way? Just as a failure to recognise the self-limiting nature of viral illnesses is a major contributory factor to the overuse of antibiotics, shouldn't we recognise inappropriate medicalisation as a major factor in the malignant hypertrophy of medical control?

We should be encouraging a societal debate about the proper limits to medicine's domain. We should not pursue the problematisation of normality that is currently extending medicine's control over the healthy.

References

1 Illich I, 1976. Medical nemesis: The expropriation of health. London: Marion Boyars Publishers. Reissued 1995 in an enlarged edition as: Limits to medicine. London: Marion Boyars.
2 Skrabanek P, 1994. The death of humane medicine and the rise of coercive healthism. London: The Social Affairs Unit.
3 Freymann J, 1994, quoted in Meador C. The last well person. New England Journal of Medicine; 330: 440–1.
4 Meador C, 1994. The last well person. New England Journal of Medicine; 330: 440–1.
5 Paykel E and Priest R, 1992. Recognition and management of depression in general practice:

consensus statement. BMJ; 305: 1198–202.

6 Dowrick C and Buchan I, 1995. Twelve month outcome of depression in general practice: does detection or disclosure make a difference? BMJ; 311: 1274–6.

7 Beck A et al, 1961. An inventory for measuring depression. Archives of General Psychiatry; 4: 561–71.

8 Hamilton M, 1960. A rating scale for depression. Journal of Neurological and Neurosurgical Psychiatry; 23: 59–61.

9 Heath I, 1999. Commentary: There must be limits to the medicalisation of human distress. BMJ; 318: 439–40.5 Frame P and Carlson S, 1975. A critical review of periodic health screening criteria, Part 4. Journal of Family Practice: 2.

10 McWhinney I, 1981. A textbook of family medicine. Oxford: Oxford University Press.

11 Hart J, 1993. Hypertension, Community control of high blood pressure. 3rd edition. Oxford: Radcliffe Medical Press.

12 Haynes R et al, 1978. Increased absenteeism from work after detection and labelling of hypertensive patients. New England Journal of Medicine; 299: 741–4.

13 Jachuck S et al, 1982. The effect of hypotensive drugs of the quality of life. Journal of the Royal College of General Practitioners; 32: 103–5.

14 Marteau T, 1989. Psychological costs of screening. BMJ; 299: 527.

15 Marteau T, 1990. Reducing the psychological costs. BMJ; 301: 26–8.

16 Totman R, 1990. Mind, stress and health. London: Souvenir Press.

17 Hart J, 1971. The inverse care law. Lancet; i: 405–12.

18 Wilson J, Jungner G, 1968. Principle and practice of screening for disease. WHO Public Health Paper no 34. Geneva: WHO.

19 Davey Smith G, Egger M 1994. Who benefits from medical interventions? Editorial, BMJ; 308: 72–4.

20 Armstrong D, 1995. The rise of surveillance medicine. Sociology of Health & Illness; 17, 3: 393–404.

21 Foucault M, 1974. Birth of the clinic. An archaeology of medical perception. London: Tavistock Publications. Foucault is not easy to read, but always brings a fresh perspective – it is worth the struggle.

22 Armstrong D, 1995: The rise of surveillance medicine. Sociology of Health and Illness; 3: 393–404.

23 Popper K, 1945. The open society and its enemies. London: Routledge. Revised edition, 1950, Princeton University Press. One of the key political texts of the 20th century.

24 Shaw, G B, 1911. The Doctor's Dilemma, Act 1.

25 Wilmshurst P, 2000. Devaluing clinical skills. Personal view. BMJ; 320: 1739.

26 Freidson E, 1985. The reorganisation of the medical profession. Medical Care Review; 42: 11–35.

27 Berlant J, 1975. Profession and monopoly. Berkekey: University of California Press.

28 Starr P, 1982. The social transformation of American medicine. New York: Basic Books.

29 Illich I, 1976. Medical nemesis: The expropriation of health. London: Marion Boyars Publishers. Reissued 1995 in an enlarged edition as: Limits to medicine. London: Marion Boyars.

30 Holloway G, 1994. Susto and the career path of the victim of an industrial accident: a sociological case study. Social Science and Medicine; 38: 989–97.

31 Illich I, 1976. Medical nemesis: The expropriation of health. London: Marion Boyars Publishers. Reissued 1995 in an enlarged edition as: Limits to medicine. London: Marion Boyars. Chap 2.

32 Eastman N, 1999. Public health psychiatry or crime prevention? BMJ; 318: 549–51.

33 The Sleep Council, 1998. Magazine advertisement.

34 "PM" programme, BBC Radio 4, 11 May 1998.

35 Kubler-Ross E, 1969. On death and dying. New York: Macmillan.

36 de Beauvoir S, 1969. A very easy death. London: Penguin.

37 John Stuart Mill, 1859. On Liberty. Reissued 1985, London: Penguin Classics.

38 Marmot M et al, 1997. Contribution of job control and other risk factors to social variations in coronary heart disease incidence. Lancet; 350: 235–9.

8 Anthropological models

Formerly, when religion was strong and science weak, men mistook magic for medicine, now, when science is strong and religion weak, men mistake medicine for magic.

Thomas Szasz, 1973. The Second Sin

The central ethical problem in medicine is the responsible use of power.

Howard Brody, 1992. The Healer's Power

They ... thought that everything was still possible for them; which presupposed that pestilences were impossible. They fancied themselves free, and no one will ever be free so long as there are pestilences.

Albert Camus. The Plague, 1947.

Chapter summary

We may find paternalism problematic, but it won't go away. Patients sometimes want us to be paternalistic. We are cast into a role within society that in other cultures would be filled by a shaman.

Why Dr Findlay wouldn't die

An elderly man came to see me. Walking through the door he exclaimed, "You're not going to be very pleased with me." He had stopped his medication because of side effects. I explained that was fine, and we discussed what to do next. At the end of the consultation I asked him how he had thought I would react. He told me that he was relieved not to be told off as he had been by his previous doctor. He added "Of course I'm going back years ago to when doctors were doctors."

My first thought was to congratulate myself on my enlightened consulting style. Then I realised that I was reacting as if he had said, "I'm going back years ago, to when doctors were grumpy and controlling." What he actually said then hit me: "...to when doctors were doctors." I began to reflect on the implications of his statement. In what way had I failed to behave as a proper doctor?

This chapter looks at the Dr Findlay problem, the issue of paternalism. Or to be more specific, at patients' expectation of paternalism. We may deride it but it won't go away. Why? I believe my patient elegantly expressed the reason. We are not the only stakeholders fighting over the doctor's role. Society has a right to co-define our role, with our approval or without.

Richard Savage, in a remarkable randomised controlled study, showed that patients were more satisfied with the doctor consulting in a paternalistic style rather than a sharing style.[1] This was particularly striking for patients presenting with physical problems. When patients are sick they want us to tell them what to do about it. This particular finding has recently been confirmed by McKinstry, who also found that the elderly particularly favoured a doctor-directed style.[2]

It is ironic that, in exploring the agenda of the patient (an adult–adult transaction), there can be an inherent tension with the agenda of the patient (a parent–child transaction). One could construct this as a paradox – a sharing non-paternalistic consulting style can be established only by a doctor paternalistically imposing it.

Paternalism literally means to act as a father. It means to act in an authoritative way, making decisions about the patient without reference to their own choices, but with the intention to act for their good. Remember though that our ways are not inherent or immutable. The idea of paternalism as something to be analysed critically only dates back a little over two centuries. Kant criticised the paternalism of governments, saying that it "cancels freedom".[3] Previously in Western culture there was a more automatic acceptance of an authority structure throughout society. Autonomy, as we understand it, is a new-fangled Western idea, and in my opinion a jolly good one.

The standard contemporary Western system of medical ethics relies on balancing four principles:[4]

Beneficence: doing good – acting to improve the patient's health
Non-maleficence: avoiding harm to the patient
Autonomy: respecting the patient's choices and making those choices real
Justice: giving the patient their due and balancing that with the needs of others.

Paternalism therefore tends to contradict the principle of autonomy. It implies the doctor seizing the decision-making process from the patient, dispensing with informed consent and patient choice. However in reality it's not black and white. There are a number of areas where paternalism is OK. They all relate to the limits of autonomy. Autonomy presupposes that the patient is able to understand the nature and consequences of his choices. (This is not contingent on them choosing what you think is best!) A patient lacks the capacity for autonomy if they are unconscious or psychotic. In this situation medical paternalism is seen as an appropriate response that should act to protect the patient's best interest.

In the case of a young child, of course, autonomy resides with the parent. As the child grows there is a grey area where autonomy gradually transfers to the child. The "Gillick rules" are a helpful response to one example of this dilemma.[5,6] But the principles behind the Gillick rules don't always give me a clear answer. What about the ten-year-old child who clearly doesn't want a travel vaccine that his parent insists he must have?

The fringes of autonomy

Paternalism is one of those awkward areas in medicine. We're not supposed to approve of it, but it's not always bad. We can cope with tightly controlled paternalism such as dispensing with fully informed consent in an emergency or in the case of those incapable of exercising genuine autonomy due to psychotic illness or unconsciousness. We can cope with the sweet old lady who exercises her autonomy by saying, "I'll do whatever you suggest doctor."

The common problems in my own practice are those of time, and of how far to go with autonomy. If I am pressured for time the easy option is to dominate the consultation a little more, smile a little wider, talk a little louder, control the management a little more, and close things down sooner. I'm sure I could devise a measure that proved I was being more efficient, but this is commonplace paternalism, and I don't like it.

My other dilemma is how far to go before I can call it autonomy. Imagine the doctor checking out every possibility with a patient with a urinary tract infection:

"We could leave it to see if it resolves or I could treat you now?

"OK, would you prefer Trimethoprim which is a cheap tablet, so that will help you to feel you are freeing NHS resources for other patients, or you could have Cefadroxil which costs a bit more and is slightly more likely to work first time but also slightly more likely to give you thrush?

"Now, a three-day course is standard, but Jones showed that a single dose works nearly as well, or you could opt for the old fashioned five-day course?

"And would you prefer them blister packed or in a bottle?

"Oh, and which lab did you want me to send the MSU off to?

"Run screaming from the room? – Yes, I guess that's a valid choice."

The answer of course is, I need to check out as much as the patient wants me to check out. But logically I can only be sure of that by checking everything out. Therefore I use my own judgement. That's paternalism. And I guess this sort of "common sense paternalism" is part of my job.

But just like medicalisation, generating paternalism is not the sole province of the doctor. The focus of this chapter is on the paternalism that is sought by patients, such as my elderly man at the beginning of the chapter.

Charles Fried states that the doctor is "the servant, not of life in the abstract, but of the life plan of the patient".[7] Respect for autonomy does not remove the problem of the doctor's power. We still have the power to determine how we analyse the patient's problem, what choices we offer, and what spin we put on those choices.

Rather than pretend that these choices are not open to us, Fried suggests that we should modify our choices to serve the life plan of the patient. Let us then explore what this means.

The shamanistic role of the doctor

Helman, a medical anthropologist, points out that there are common human behaviours operating within any culturally defined healing system, whether you are a Western medic or a third-world shaman.[8] Forget the content of Western medicine for a moment and consider the process of consulting a healer:

Shaman	Western medic
Consultation process moulded by local cultural expectations	Consultation process moulded by local cultural expectations
Tribal authority figure	Tribal authority figure
Distinctive appearance with special clothes and personal markings indicating seniority	Distinctive appearance with white coat, name badge and optional stethoscope round neck (junior) or Mercedes (senior)
Given responsibility for defining who is sick	Given responsibility for defining who is sick
Takes a holistic approach to the sick patient	Takes a holistic approach to the sick patient?
Uses secretly learned rituals to come to a diagnosis	Uses methods learned at medical school to come to a diagnosis
Uses loud dramatic rituals in difficult cases	Uses MRI scanner in difficult cases
May consult with mysterious and remote others such as spirit guides or ancestors	May consult with mysterious and remote others such as teaching hospital consultants
Uses ritual objects such as bones, feathers and rattles	Uses ritual objects such as stethoscope, prescription pad and pill bottles
Gives medication with detailed instructions of how to use it	Gives medication with pack insert
Takes over responsibility for the cure of the patient's illness	Takes over responsibility for the cure of the patient's illness

I am not saying ground-up beetles and herbs are an equally effective treatment for pneumonia as amoxicillin. I am saying that the process of obtaining the ground-up beetles and herbs serves the same social function as the process of obtaining the amoxicillin.

The pre-test probability of pathology needing antibiotics in a healthy afebrile young man with a three-day history of productive cough who is breathing normally is close to zero. Why then do I listen to his chest? For exactly the same reason that the shaman rattles his bones. It fulfils a social function and contains powerful medicine. It makes for a happy patient who knows he has offloaded the uncertainty of his illness onto the shoulders of the professional.

Like the shaman our role is determined in part by our culture. Payer examined differences in the health cultures between the USA and Europe.[9] She found that the USA reported higher rates of various different types of surgery, reflecting a model of the body as a machine that needs overhauling and repairing. Surgery was also more aggressive, and drug doses were often higher, reflecting an assertive "fix it" attitude.

In the majority of doctor–patient encounters there are no critical biomedical interventions which, if muffed, would lead to great harm to the patient. (There is a minority of encounters of course that are critical – I am not saying medicine is useless. Furthermore in any consultation there is the possibility of iatrogenic harm.) Why then do patients come to doctors so often?

Our patients seek from us the same thing as people in other cultures seek from their shamans. All around the world there are formalised "folk healers" such as shamans, herb doctors, mambos, isangomas, sahis.[10] The term "shaman" is often used as a generic term, including the concept of "healer" and "priest". A shaman is seen as having two functions. He acts as an authority figure who takes responsibility for the patient's illness. He is also seen as someone possessing special, often supernatural, powers, not held by others.

The shaman's role provides members of the social group with a very powerful coping strategy. The shaman provides socially sanctioned ego defences that help the patient:

- They enable the patient to reduce his level of fear on facing illness.
- They lessen the psychological burden of future uncertainty.
- They provide a structure for what to do when he is ill.
- They put the ill person in a socially defined role so that other will. support him.
- They provide hope because of the shaman's special powers

If you consider what is known about the psychology of illness then these benefits can be seen as very real. Consider the role of the shaman in helping the patient to perform Moos and Schaefer's seven illness tasks described in Chapter 4.[11]

I am not considering the claims of some shaman to possess supernatural power or experience any sort of spiritual encounter. That is an issue that lies beyond this work and is a red herring with respect to my thesis. I am looking at the social role of the shaman, and asking what is going on between the players in the setting of their cultural expectations. Within a Western setting we might see it as a priestly role. We are cast as the priests of our secularised society.

The ultimate anthropological proof that we are the shamans of the West comes from the sahis, the local folk healers in the Raymah area of Yemen.[12] With no formal training they inject into their patients whatever Western drugs they have. Interestingly they use less of a holistic/counselling approach than other types of shaman, as the injections themselves are seen as possessing great potency (they're good enough for rich Westerners after all.) Given that few of our patients will read the data sheet, can we say there is no shamanistic element to medication seeking behaviour in the West?

Ontological assault?

I am happy to be grown up and choose my own way when things go well. But when illness or misfortune strikes, behaviour patterns may regress.[13] Pellegrino describes illness as an "ontological assault".[14] This phrase has a teasing ambiguity. Illness is a threat felt at the deepest level of self, and illness is also a threat to the survival of the self.

As adults we accept a fair amount of uncertainty in our lives (will I get a bonus / will my child get a good report / will Crystal Palace get back into the Premiership?). I may reduce excessive stresses or threats to my psyche either by unloading responsibility for them onto someone else, or by demanding a childish yes/no response to my uncertainty.

The issue then is what constitutes an "excessive" stress or threat? I don't know the answer to that. I know that when my neighbour needed his car push-starting one day I felt happy to help, but if he wanted me to do it once a week because he habitually left his lights on I might not be so keen. What is a "reasonable" load for an individual to bear?

St Paul gave a paradoxical guideline in his letter to the Galatians: "Carry each other's burdens, and in this way you will fulfil the law of Christ ... Each one should test his own actions. Then he can take pride in himself, without comparing himself to somebody else, for each one should carry his own load".[15] Carry each other's burdens but each one should carry his own load. This is pretty good advice for contemporary Western society. The only difficulty is in telling the difference between the two. What is an unreasonable burden that needs help from others, and what load should I just bear and get on with? What is certain is that when someone's load becomes too burdensome, some of it may get presented to us.

Magical thinking

We may not like to mix our medicine with magic, but the age of reason still finds room for magical thinking – at least the National Lottery shows no signs of imminent bankruptcy. The logical response to the Lottery is not to buy a ticket, but millions do. "Logic" is not the way human thinking works. We don't just think about the odds. Davison found that notions of "luck, fate and destiny" were integral to a lay understanding of disease causation.[16] We believe that we are special, and that our life holds a particular importance. Why we should believe such a thing is interesting, but I must leave issues of meaning to another debate.

Given that magical thinking is alive and well, the tribal shaman is surely its most natural focus. It is sometimes hard to tell where therapeutic naivety ends and magical thinking begins. Earlier today one of my partners de-briefed from a taxing consultation with a young mother who announced that her toddler had eaten "nothing but sweets for the last three weeks". Whilst the toddler happily demolished my partner's consulting room, any attempt to engage with the mother about ways of modifying behaviour were met with overt dissatisfaction. The child's preference for sweets was seen as a problem to be "fixed", and the mother was beginning to get pretty fed up with my partner talking rather than acting. Where there is an external locus of control located in a "powerful other" then the patient will appoint us as tribal shaman with full trimmings. It's what we're paid for.

Practical shamanism

Some doctors set out to be shamans, but most of us have shamanism thrust upon us. Balint pointed out that the doctor is himself a powerful drug.[17] We assume that the patient has come for a medical answer, but often they come for a therapeutic transaction.

The shaman has a number of parental tasks. I have divided them into the benign and the dysfunctional. The distinction is not a clear one, but relates to whether on balance the parental role expected of the doctor can be seen as a "reasonable" ego defence mechanism or as an "unreasonable" regressive activity. Yes, I agree it's as reliable as predicting the weather, but make your own judgement on these cases.

Benign shamanism

It is possible to define a number of categories where doctors behave in a way which is paternalistic, culturally defined and arguably is in the patients' best interest. (I am excluding those categories such as acute major trauma and psychosis where autonomy is unrealisable.)

Parental support

Case report

Julie is an older teenager. At her birthday party her father was seriously assaulted by an acquaintance, which sparked off a series of interpersonal and interfamily problems.

Her family network is strong, normally exercising an internal locus of control within the group. This problem, and Julie's reaction to it, overwhelmed their normal support mechanisms. Julie exhibited a "normal" transitional reaction with some borderline depressive features. Another family member had previously required treatment with antidepressants. Her mum brought Julie to surgery, requesting antidepressants.

Here medication is seen as an "answer" to a psychosocial situation that was perceived as out of control, in the sense that the family felt unable to cope with it. Would you prescribe antidepressants? I don't think there is a right or wrong answer – I think what would make an answer better or worse is how you prescribe or don't prescribe.

I felt that the normally successful parenting capacity of the family had broken down, and they were asking me to lend myself as a parent whilst they recovered. Perhaps it was because of their recognition that the parental role normally belonged to them that the request was to lend this parenting in an explicitly medical way – as a tablet. If I was a better doctor I would have boosted the family's own parenting capacity with a timely psychological intervention. But I also felt inclined to respond in the way that the family, with Julie's full approval, had decided for themselves was best.

I prescribed. Julie rapidly got better, more quickly than could be expected given the mechanism of action of antidepressants. The family regained a sense of control. I stopped the medication long before the proper guidelines tell me to, and all remains well.

Sometimes we can offer parental support without even knowing it. A 68-year-old lady saw me for some routine reason. I took the opportunity to ask her how she was getting on following her lumpectomy, radiotherapy and tamoxifen for her breast carcinoma diagnosed a couple of years previously. Her reply fascinated me. She said, "With your support I'm doing OK... I always say with my GP's support I'm OK..." When I checked her records I saw that she had only seen me three times since her surgery, and yet her perception was that we had helped to bear her burden.

It has always been seen as part of the doctor's role to offer human support to the patient. When I become ill I do not want a biotechnician who gives me evidence-based injections but doesn't help me to face my fears. In dealing with severe distress or terminal illness we are taught the role (and the perils) of touching the patient. It confirms our presence as a human support as well as a medical technician. To offer human support to someone in distress seems to me to be a parental act. Our challenge is to offer this parenting in an appropriate and controlled way.

Parental permission

Case report

Gwen is 75 years old, fit as a fiddle and still a keen dancer. She presented with a DVT for which I admitted her. She initially mobilised on a Zimmer frame. Her anticoagulation was well controlled by the Haematologists and she was mobilising steadily. I encouraged her to gradually increase her level of activity.

She was concerned as to exactly how quickly she should increase her walking, and was clearly unhappy with just going at her own pace. She said, "I don't want to do anything wrong – I'll follow your instructions."

I therefore agreed to review her a few times to observe her walking – a bit better each time – and duly congratulated her on her progress.

Gwen puzzled me. She is intelligent and has reasonable social support, but she needed me to be there with the water wings even when she had learned to swim. She also has a rather old-fashioned view of the world: "I don't want to do anything wrong". I therefore gave a "medical structure" to her natural recovery. I had to give her permission to get better.

Priestly magic

Case report

Donna is a young lady who has had anterior knee pain for three months. It irritates her and interferes with climbing too many stairs but does not limit her in any other way. She is otherwise healthy with no history of injury. On examination there is a minor degree of tenderness on patella pressure, otherwise the knee is entirely normal.

The biomedical viewpoint is that the problem is likely to settle and that intervention would be unlikely to change anything. This viewpoint did not prove popular. A more acceptable formula was to send her for an X-ray (her plan) and then to simply observe (my plan).

X-rays still retain magic power. Better still are "scans" (it doesn't matter scanning what with what). An MRI is a powerful rattling of bones (the fact that it sounds like it's rattling something heavy and expensive inside helps).

Many of the things we do have the same social functioning as the shaman's rattling of bones over his patient. Many of our interventions lack reliable evidence of real benefit. Consider:

- Antibiotics for simple otitis media.
- Tepid sponging for fever.
- "Routine" physiotherapy after rheumatology or orthopaedic assessment.

Health service managers look askance at some of our practices, and yet the patients keep on coming back. They come because it's not about evidence, it's about medicine. It's about being given coping mechanisms in a scary world. It is not for us as a separate tribe to deny culturally normative magic to the lay majority. It is for us to negotiate with the tribe as a whole the reasonable limits of our role.

We are all trapped by our own magic. A tribal shaman cannot say to his heartsink: "This will get better on its own." He has to rattle the bones.

I remember my sense of confusion during my house officer induction day. A microbiologist gave us a brief pep talk. Three years earlier he had drummed into us that we should never start a course of antibiotics without sending a sample to the lab ("like those dreadful GPs do"). Now, when we were housemen, he emptied a big box of old lab forms onto the table and said, "each one of these represents a £1 note". (My, it *was* a long time ago.) "Why do housemen request so many useless tests? Send less tests, we have to save money." I wanted to say "but you said to us…", but housemen didn't ask too many questions in 1979.

Priestly rites

Case report

Mr J was an older man from an ethnic minority community. He died at home after a brief and stormy struggle with bowel cancer. He died uncomplaining, supported by his wife and children with our Hospice's homecare team monitoring in the background. The strength of this family made me realise how much I was used to us as medics being the driving force in the care of the dying patient. I saw Mr J before and just after death, and told the family I would return to give the death certificate.

I returned at lunchtime. I was greeted with great courtesy by the oldest son and sat with the family in the front room. We talked about Mr J's life, and about his death, and I produced the book of death certificates. The room went quiet as I filled in the certificate. I realised I was filling in ritual phrases – "Ia: carcinomatosis. Ib: carcinoma of the colon." I confirmed my priestly credentials by filling in the letters after my name "as registered by the GMC". This was a final rite of passage, marking Mr J's release from his suffering. It was a rite as solemn as any Mass.

The social function of a priest or shaman involves creating ritual that enables the patient to deal with the numinous – the sense of the mystery that lies beyond our own experience. We can be protected from the mystery beyond us by the routine of life and also by the West's dominant religion of materialism. Suffering and fear puncture these defences. Now that the west has marginalised religious priests it finds it needs secular ones. We've been voted in.

Priestly appeasement

Case report

Jean is in her 40s. She attends because two members of her family have died from carcinoma of the pancreas. Her sister in the USA has had an ultrasound scan to "check" that she doesn't have carcinoma of the pancreas. Jean, very understandably, would like an ultrasound scan too. She is asymptomatic.

Imaging her pancreas is very unlikely to be an effective way of intercepting an early carcinoma. Carcinoma of the pancreas is renowned for its rapid growth, and an ultrasound is not good at detecting very small deep tumours. So if she developed a carcinoma of the pancreas how long would it be between being detectable by ultrasound and being symptomatic? In the absence of prospective trial evidence your guess is as good as mine. My guess was that it may need to be repeated every few months in order to have any meaning as a screening procedure, and that I did not think that trials with a screening group of one were a very good idea.

Feeling a heel, I tried to discuss some of these issues with her (will I never learn?). She of course still wanted a scan, and I, of course, sent her for one. I also sent her for the opinion of our very sensible local biliary-pancreatic surgeon, who had a pretty similar discussion with her, albeit with a few more facts up his sleeve. Jean was reassured by her normal scan and has not pressed me for a repeat after a period of two years.

Health-seeking behaviour is usually reasonable (having a reason) but is not always logical. I realised that Jean's scan was a way for her to cope with the fear of thinking about a new threat. It had enabled her to appease fate and then move on.

Consider the number needed to treat (NNT) to prevent one bad outcome for most screening interventions. Why do all these people agree to be screened? Partly because we tend to feed them benefit figures based on a relative risk reduction model. But also because it is our modern equivalent to a votive offering brought by penitents to the temple of Hygeia. It is a psychological trick to manage our fear of disease.

Dysfunctional shamanism

The search for paternalism may sometimes be justified, serving a legitimate social function. There again, sometimes it may not. There are inappropriate bids for paternalism, which come from an unhealthy desire for dependency.

Primary dependency (medicalisation – see Chapter 7)

Case report

Chloe's records are as thick as a doorstop, but her summary card is sparsely marked with just one overdose and three normal deliveries. She consults about herself. She consults about her kids. She consults because she is tired. She consults because she cannot cope. Let's face it, she just consults.

Her relationship with her partner is destructive but persistent. Any attempt by myself or the counsellors to deal with underlying issues seems to run straight down the drain. One day she says "I've been given one lot of counselling at the [mental health advice] centre, and they're going to give me some more."

Chloe is not using us as a source of help. She is using us as a source of legitimisation for her role as a victim. Her conceptualisation of counselling fascinated me – "I've been given one lot of counselling…" Counselling is seen as a therapeutic substance to be administered by a powerful other. She's been given two kilograms of it this week, and she's coming back to get three kilograms more. She constructs her problem as a failure of this therapeutic substance to resolve her difficulties.

There are two ways of looking at this. One could say that we offer her support – a friendly face in a bleak life. What chance is there for a poorly-supported mum on a council estate? Her conceptualisation of herself as a passive agent who bears no responsibility for her misery is a realistic ego defence.

Or one could say that, in consenting to medicalise problems that we cannot possibly solve for her, we are responsible for her never taking responsibility for them herself. Her only chance of growth and change is to napalm the surgery and get on with her life. (Actually, some of the local youths are working on that!)

Secondary dependency (post knight-in-shining-armour syndrome)

Case report

Fred is now in his 80s, but nearly didn't make it. He seldom consulted, but presented with worsening prostatism in his mid-70s. I referred him to a Urologist. He joined the waiting list for a TURP. After a few months his urinary stream deteriorated and I wrote to the urologist to see if his surgery could be expedited. The months went by.

Fred's wife phoned me towards the end of a Friday evening surgery. She sounded anxious. Fred was having difficulty in breathing, but had been trying not to make a fuss. I visited, and found him to be in gross heart failure and chronic urinary retention. I admitted him. He had an obstructive uropathy causing acute renal failure, finally presenting in heart failure. After a prolonged and stormy admission his ARF settled, and his heart failure responded well to medical treatment.

He got his TURP and made a gradual recovery. He and his wife needed intensive follow up, to monitor his heart failure and his electrolytes, and also to help him regain confidence after what he found to be a psychologically shattering experience. (I remember the intense discussions about the potassium content of every available edible vegetable.) I was "a tower of strength" and helped pull them through.

Fred is now as fit as a fiddle. His creatinine remains steady in the low two hundreds. We check his cardiovascular system and his renal function twice a year. The only trouble is that not a month goes by that this healthy couple doesn't see me at least twice. I have become the arbiter of every minor malaise or social hiccup. I've tried to talk them out of it but their smiling faces still appear, keen to see "their doctor", who "saved Fred's life".

I offered support, as a strong expert who would help to see them through a crisis. I feel, even in retrospect, that the support I offered was appropriate. The offer was accepted with both hands, and not relinquished once the crisis ceased. My intervention transformed these patients from self-reliance to dependency. In Fred's case this was complicated by the "oh crikey" syndrome (a term I use since a patient said those words to me in this context.) The "oh crikey" syndrome is characterised by an increased sense of vulnerability, triggered by minor symptoms, following a major health threat.

I have seen a similar inappropriate persistence of dependence after other crises. Bereavements are a common trigger, perhaps because the doctor is also a link with the one who is lost. Just like primary dependence the effect is to reduce the patient's self-reliance, and thus reduce their own ability to grow and make their own choices in life.

Even appropriate support is a potent drug whose side effects and addictive potential cannot be ignored.

Induced dependency

Case report

As this is a game one is generally blind to I will have to report someone else's case. (I'll leave it to them to report one of mine.)

Dr F, despite the availability of community networks and a local Citizens' Advice Bureau, often filled in DSS benefit application forms for her patients if they found them too complicated. (It was surprising how many of her patients began to find them too complicated.) She would always collect housebound patients' prescriptions from the pharmacist herself, and she was not above doing the odd spot of shopping for them too.

Dr F had an ever enlarging band of followers within her practice. She was greatly missed when she left the practice suddenly due to a breakdown of her mental health.

There's enough demand for parenting out there without us offering more. Induced dependency may be due to a doctor's naivety, misunderstanding what makes a "good" doctor. It is far more likely to be due to personality traits in the doctor which, in reality, get in the way of them being an effective doctor. This issue was discussed in Chapter 3.

Practising safe shamanism

So what determines when (or how far) medical paternalism is OK? If we ignore the minor "common sense paternalism" I mention at the start of this chapter, what about the rest?

William Perry describes a map of human development (commonly known as "Perry's line").[18] He describes nine positions of personal growth. The journey starts from a childish belief that authoritative others know what is right and wrong, and all will be well if we do as we are told. The maturing adult goes through transitions involving the acceptance of complexity and the rejection of absolutisms and unquestioned authority. The mature individual may finally reach a position of commitment to his own values and choices, whilst respecting the different values and choices of others and remaining ever ready to learn. The mature individual attains full autonomy.

How should we be towards those who have never grown far along this line, such as those who are emotionally immature or damaged or threatened by suffering? If we are grown up we have attained that, at least in some part, by being parented. There is a role for us to offer some measure of parenting, some shamanism, to the vulnerable. But, like any potent drug, we must offer it appropriately. We must recognise its side effects and addictive potential. Our goal must remain progression towards an adult–adult relationship.

We are more ready to offer toxic drugs for more serious conditions. We are prepared to give vincristine for cancer. If it were found to reduce the duration of the common cold it would be unlikely to receive an extension of its product licence for this condition. The unstable drug of benign paternalism may be justified where the patient is vulnerable due to the threat of serious illness or poverty of personal development. And a diluted mixture of "common sense paternalism" is a necessary lubricant for everyday practice.

Is there not a tension between our shamanistic role and our goal for patient autonomy? Yes, certainly. But we manage many tensions in the practice of medicine, and this is one that we will manage best if we acknowledge it and reflect on how it works.

Realism, accountability, purposiveness

Ladd discussed the problem of power in the *Lancet* in 1980. He suggested there are three issues that determine whether our use of power is responsible and reasonable:

> *Realism* – being aware of the true consequences of one's acts or omissions.
> *Accountability* – being prepared to give an explanation of one's use of power.
> *Purposiveness* – having a specific goal which benefits the patient.

Ladd makes the point that we cannot share power with the patient until we acknowledge that we possess it in the first place.

When doctors were doctors

Our picture of an old-fashioned doctor might include behaviours such as:

- Paternalism
- Prescribing antibiotics for URTIs
- Prescribing cough medicines
- Giving B12 injections for tiredness
- Prescribing tranquillisers to the anxious
- Prescribing sleeping pills on request
- Prescribing a pill for every ill.

We are more enlightened. We support autonomy. We reserve antibiotics for those who need them. We rarely prescribe benzodiazepines. It's all pure science and over-the-counter paracetamol. This is biomedically appropriate, but it leaves some patients out in the cold.[19] The majority of patients attend with symptoms of illness rather than disease processes. They come seeking coping mechanisms. All we have left in our doctor's bags are potent drugs designed for diseases. We have nothing left for illness. We have to ask whether the pendulum has swung too far.

Eric Caines is a former NHS personnel director who pressed for the demystification and rationalisation of the medical profession in the 1980s. In an intriguing article in the BMA News Review entitled "Patients must never stop trusting doctors", he questions the wisdom of his former views.[20] He quotes a colleague's view that "the efficacy of the medical profession is based on myth and if you destroy the myth, you destroy the profession. Medicine is the most inexact of sciences – medicine practised by one generation of doctors exposes the inadequacies of the medicine practised by all their predecessors ... Dependency expects certainty but nothing is certain about medicine. The relationship between a patient and a doctor is, therefore, founded in mutual pretence – on a myth." Caines concludes: "When I consult a doctor, I want to be able to put myself in their hands unquestioningly. I don't want to have to make a layman's assessment of their professional capacities. I just want them to make me better and once I cease to trust in their ability to do that, my whole security is undermined. Things have gone too far and its time to change the tone of the debate."

If not us, then who?

If we no longer see ourselves as society's shamans, do we think that people will just grow up and change hard wired folk thinking into modernistic scientific thinking? (Don't we know that modernistic scientific thinking needs a facelift anyway in a postmodern age?)

We may have revolutionised medical ethics and medical practice over the last generation, but there is little evidence that the project is winning votes. Instead we are seeing a massive rise in benign quackery in the form of complementary medicine.[21] Astin found that there were more visits to complementary practitioners than to primary care physicians in the USA.[22] Patients complain of a lack of time with their GP, and of a lack of compassion.[23,24] White found that patients reported psychological benefits such as optimism and hope from the support given by complementary practitioners.[25] This increased, rather than decreased, the patient's sense of control, therefore White's paper does not support the view that such shamanism necessarily increases dependency.

My personal view is that most complementary medical systems work by a placebo effect. But then if we could develop a pill as powerful as a placebo we would win the Nobel Prize. For these sorts of placebo therapies to work their practitioners have to be excellent shamans. They give the patient time, attention and care. They seek a holistic model that includes other parts of the patient's life. They then prescribe a magic medicine in a ritualistic setting. They are traditional folk healers who are thriving in the shadow of our own shamanistic impotence.

So what is our way forward? Should we stick firmly to the ever-changing science or should we return to the days of Dr Findlay? Should we seek to become Western shamans – magician scientists? Paterson and Peacock suggest that we could actively create a more mixed marketplace of health care, integrating complementary practitioners into the primary healthcare team.[26] Dixon and Sweeney have made a bold contribution with their book "The human effect in medicine".[27] They "challenge the dogma of modern technological medicine that ignores both the therapeutic effect of the doctor and the self-healing powers of the patient". They ask whether the doctor as a physician healer could harness self-healing mechanisms within the patient's own body and mind.

Perhaps Dixon and Sweeney are suggesting a good British compromise. Can we not recognise peoples' needs in a broader way, and be prepared to split the difference? Can we not find a way of practising medicine that shows a greater respect for the culture of which we are a part?

Looking at a Co-op shift

So what difference does all this make? If we extend our gaze beyond the biomedical, if we use words and models from the broader perspectives we have examined, how does this affect our job? The doctor's shamanistic role within this broader gaze is illustrated by looking at an out-of-hours shift. In setting the scene I will mention the biomedical issues but not dwell on them. I am asking two questions:

- What's going on?
- What does the patient need from the consultation?

The practice to which I belong is covered out-of-hours by a large GP Co-op. I generally do a Sunday evening mobile shift, being driven round to calls that a colleague at base has passed on for a visit. Sunday evening is the time that things fray at the edges if you're sick. You might have been sick all weekend, hanging on for Monday when surgery re-opens, but as night draws in you can't make it. You need a doctor tonight.

This is an anonymised version of one Sunday evening shift in winter. I have changed details to protect patient identities, but even if the colours are different the patterns are true. As the shift went by it struck me just how little of what I was doing was "medical", so given that I was doing something, I noted the cases to try to work out what that something was.

Call 1

We started to drive to what eventually became call 2, but base diverted us, en route, to an urgent call to a man with difficulty breathing. The London Ambulance Service (LAS) were already on scene. Their message read "61-year old-man, possibly dying, ?LVF, but won't go to hospital". On our arrival LAS had nebulised him and he was "much better". He lived in sheltered accommodation. He had established COPD with asthma, and looked nearer 80. He was surrounded by empty lager cans and well used ashtrays.

On examination there was no LVF. He wouldn't go into hospital, as he would not be allowed alcohol or cigarettes. I started him on prednisolone – he already had some in hand. The warden came by and promised to keep an eye on him. I liked the warden - he looked like a wrestler and got on with the patient in an amiable and common sense sort of way.

- **What's going on?**
  The patient has a chronic illness, now irreversible, largely caused by smoking. He had a severe asthmatic exacerbation that was successfully treated by LAS. LAS are anxious that he is alone. He is anxious to maintain control over himself, and maintain his chosen lifestyle.

- **What do they need from the consultation?**
  LAS needed permission to leave him. They all needed me, as an

authority figure, to adjudicate. He needed permission to start the treatment he already had. My role was as an adviser and social arbiter.

Call 2

An 87-year-old woman in sheltered accommodation. She has recurrent cellulitis of the leg, threatening to break down. The warden was concerned about the possibility of "a clot". On examination the problem appeared superficial with no evidence of a DVT. The patient gets confused and takes off the dressings. A pill check shows that she is not taking her antibiotics. The warden is not allowed to administer her medication. An equally unqualified carer should give her medication, but she gets a different carer on different days. I arranged that the warden would supervise the carer.

- **What's going on?**
  A mildly confused elderly lady has chronic leg problems, with a low level of uncertainty about the possibility of a DVT, which commonly has false negative examination findings. A bureaucratic system has disempowered the warden, the person most able to manage the problem. The warden feared a reprimand if she "missed something".

- **What do they need from the consultation?**
  The warden needed me to be an authority figure, sanctioning a compromise to the bureaucratic impasse.

Call 3

Another urgent call, to a 66-year-old man with his anxious wife in their tiny old terraced house. He had just had his third ever TIA, which lasted about three minutes. There was much panic – might he be having a CVA or an MI? (He had a past history of both, and was on appropriate medication.) He calmed down with a cigarette, and was much better on our arrival. He complained of feeling shaky like "two days after action in Korea". There were no acute findings.

- **What's going on?**
  A TIA, provoking a fear of death or disability that they could not cope with.

- **What do they need from the consultation?**
  They need a shaman to tell them that "this is not the one", he will be all right.

Call 4

A teenager with his mother in a cramped attic conversion flat. He has earache after a URTI concurrent with a 14-hour plane flight. There was no OM. I advised paracetamol.

- **What's going on?**
  Self-limiting Eustachian tube obstruction, with poor parental coping mechanisms due to the lack of an adequate social support network. Desire for a magic fix to a self-limiting problem.

- **What do they need from the consultation?**
  Self-help advice from an authority figure who restores a sense of control.

Call 5

A 2-year-old with a fever. He has been on Ciprofloxacin for OM for 24 hours. The patient and his parents live in a hostile block of flats, with a Pit Bull type of dog for security in a basket by the front door. The room is hot. They are giving sub-optimal doses of paracetamol. Examination confirms OM only, and the child's general condition is satisfactory. I advise the worried parents.

- **What's going on?**
  Parental anxiety and lack of experience, exacerbated by the lack of a "granny" figure to coach and reassure. A parental desire for a magic fix to a problem that will soon resolve.

- **What do they need from the consultation?**
  Coaching and reassurance from an authority figure, as a granny is not prescribable.

Call 6

A middle-aged woman who six days previously had witnessed the failed resuscitation of her husband for haematemesis, during which he had received 10 units of blood. A neighbour had found her, confused and covered in red nail varnish. Her son was now with her, and was coping well. She has a past history of mental health problems, the son is not sure what, but it doesn't sound as if she has ever had a psychotic illness or admission. She is in a partially disassociated state, denying that her husband is dead, and is preoccupied with cleaning the house. She appears to be in no danger. I chat to the son about defence mechanisms. He will stay with her to ensure her safety, and will call us if there is further concern. I arrange for her own GP to review the situation tomorrow. This call takes some time.

- **What's going on?**
  The patient is in "hysterical" denial as an effective, albeit temporary, defence mechanism from a traumatic and horrendous loss.

- **What do they need from the consultation?**

The patient needs to be able to face the early stage of her traumatic loss at her own pace, with family support, in a secure environment. The son needs to be reassured that he has the appropriate human resources to help his mother. The son also needs a sympathetic shaman to offload on in the absence of anyone else, as he is also processing his own loss. They both need the permission and support of an authority figure to get through this with their own coping mechanisms, rather than medicalising the problem.

Call 7

A lady in her 70s with a productive cough two days after her cataract extraction. I prescribe amoxycillin.

- **What's going on?**
  A borderline bronchitis, possibly as a result of a general anaesthetic.

- **What do they need from the consultation?**
  A minor biomedical intervention and reassurance that all will be well.

Call 8

A young self-employed tradesman who has had intermittent left renal pain for five days. He is being investigated by his GP and has adequate analgesia, and is due an urgent Outpatient appointment in the week. However his girlfriend wants it sorted out now. I check him over, but there is nothing that can be done at the weekend to further his management.

- **What's going on?**
  Tolerance of uncertainty can be hard. Loss of income can be harder. A magic fix would be better.

- **What do they need from the consultation?**
  I can give a reassuring second opinion and advise patience, but I feel I have little more to offer.

Call 9

A middle-aged woman receiving chemotherapy for cancer. She has been vomiting since the last cycle two days ago, and now has dysuria and frequency. Urinalysis is suggestive of a UTI. I give her some Cefadroxil and an antiemetic. The family is extremely anxious. We spend a few minutes talking about her treatment and I listen to her fears.

- **What's going on?**
  A minor medical problem is the last straw for coping mechanisms that have been over-stretched.

- **What do they need from the consultation?**
  A minor medical fix. A shaman who can restore a sense of control and hope.

Call 10

A five-year-old girl with fever, abdominal pain and vomiting. She has a past history of UTI. On examination there is evidence of a viral throat infection only – urine was clear to dipstick. I advised paracetamol and arranged for a check MSU to go to the lab in the morning.

- **What's going on?**
  A self-limiting viral fever with an understandable parental concern because of her past history.

- **What do they need from the consultation?**
  Someone to check out their concerns and to offer support.

Call 11

An elderly man with dementia who lives with his extended family. He had been wandering the streets for an hour and a half, dressed only in a shirt and shoes, before being brought back by the police. It was the first time this had happened, and the family was very upset. He was unharmed – it had been warm for the time of year. He had cold peripheries but was otherwise well.

- **What's going on?**
  Family anxiety and guilt over their failure to be perfect carers.

- **What do they need from the consultation?**
  They needed a shaman who would say things were OK and restore the normal order.

That evening I practised very little biomedicine, but I feel that I did plenty that I would wish to be included in the job of being a doctor. Most of what I did would have been done as well or better in other societies by a neighbour, a granny, a shaman or a priest. My role was to stand in the breach for a society that either does not have – or does not use – neighbours, grannies, shaman or priests.

Conclusion

Human culture throughout time and place seems hard-wired to include the role of folk-healer or shaman, giving powerful coping mechanisms to the sick. These mechanisms may have a biologically beneficial effect. Medicine's increasing focus on biomedical fixes does not seem to have reduced peoples' need for a shaman figure. If we can no longer fulfil a shamanistic role within our culture then others will. We need to consider how we can respond to people's need for a shaman whilst retaining the benefits of the Western medical system and also our respect for autonomy.

References

1 Savage R and Armstrong D, 1990. Effect of a general practitioner's consulting style on patients' satisfaction: a controlled study. BMJ; 301: 968–70.
2 McKinstry B, 2000. Do patients wish to be involved in decision making in the consultation? A cross sectional survey with video vignettes. BMJ; 321: 867–71.
3 Immanuel Kant (1724–1804). Quoted in Beauchamp T and Childress J, 1994. Principles of biomedical ethics. Oxford: Oxford University Press. Chap 5.
4 Gillon R, 1985. Philosophical medical ethics. Chichester: John Wiley and Sons.
5 Gillick v West Norfolk and Wisbech Area Health Authority [1986] Court of Appeal Cases, 112.
6 See "Confidentiality and people under 16", 1993. London: British Medical Association, General Medical Services Committee, Health Education Authority, Brook Advisory Centres, Family Planning Association, Royal College of General Practitioners.
7 Fried C, 1974. Medical experimentation: Personal integrity and social policy. New York: American Elsevier.
8 Helman C, 1990. Culture, health and Illness. 2nd edn. Oxford: Butterworth-Heinemann. Chap 4.
9 Payer L, 1988. Medicine and culture. New York: Henry Holt.
10 Helman C, 1990. Culture, health and Illness. 2nd edn. Oxford: Butterworth-Heinemann. Chap 4.
11 Moos R and Schaefer J, 1984. The crisis of physical illness: an overview and conceptual approach. Chapter 1 in Moos R (ed.) Coping with physical illness. vol 2: New perspectives. New York: Plenum.
12 Underwood P and Underwood Z, 1981. New spells for old: expectations and realities of Western medicine in a remote tribal society in Yemen, Arabia. In: Stanley N and Joshe R (eds), Changing disease pattern and human behaviour. London: Academic Press.
13 Cassell E, 1976. The healer's art. Philadelphia: Lippincott.
14 Pellegrino E 1979. Towards a reconstruction of medical morality: the primacy of the act of profession and the fact of illness. Journal of Medicine and Philosophy; 4: 32–56.
15 Galatians Ch 6, V 2 and 5. New International Version of the Bible. London: Hodder and Stoughton.
16 Davison C, 1992. The limits of lifestyle: re-assessing 'fatalism' in the popular culture of illness prevention. Social Science and Medicine; 34: 675–85.
17 Balint M, 1957. The doctor, his patient and the illness. London: Pitman.
18 Perry W, 1985. Cognitive and ethical growth: the making of meaning. Chapter 3 in Chickering A (ed.), The modern American college. San Francisco: Jossey-Bass.
19 Baker R 1996. Characteristics of practices, general practitioners and patients related to patients' satisfaction with consultations. British Journal of General Practice; 46: 601–5.
20 Caines E, 2000. Patients must never stop trusting doctors. BMA News Review. July 8: p 47.
21 Goldbeck-Wood S, 1996. Complementary medicine is booming worldwide. BMJ; 313: 131–3.
22 Astin J 1998. Why patients use alternative medicine. JAMA; 280: 1548–53.
23 Cromarty I 1996. What do patients think about during their consultations? A qualitative study. British Journal of General Practice; 46: 525–8.
24 Taylor M, 1997. Compassion: its neglect and importance. British Journal of General Practice; 47: 521–3.
25 White P, 2000. What can general practice learn from complementary medicine? British Journal

of General Practice; 50: 821–3.

26 Paterson C and Peacock W, 1995. Complementary practitioners as part of the primary health care team: evaluation of one model. British Journsal of General Practice; 45: 225–8.

27 Dixon M and Sweeney K, 2000. The human effect in medicine. Abingdon: Radcliffe Medical Press.

9 The role of the drug

The desire to take medicine is perhaps the greatest feature which distinguishes man from animals.

Doctors should use new remedies quickly while they are still efficacious.

Both quotes: Sir William Osler, 1849–1919

Chapter summary

We may wish to see ourselves as rational prescribers, using the products of the explosion in 20th-century biotechnology as tools that target the bio-medical problems of our patients. We must recognise however that the reasons that patients take medicines stem as much from our ancestral and societal voices as from biotechnology. We need to understand both worlds.

Looking at prescribing

The power to prescribe

It should be simple – doctors prescribe medications that have been proven to work for the relevant condition, and do not prescribe those that don't. Reality is messier. In reality doctors often prescribe in ways that seem irrational:

- We prescribe drugs with little supporting evidence: e.g. antibiotics for sore throats or otitis media.[1,2,3,4,5]
- We fail to consistently prescribe drugs that have good supporting evidence: e.g. antihypertensives and anticoagulants.[6,7]
- We do not consistently change our prescribing habits as new evidence becomes available.[8,9,10]

Facts such as these drive managers and politicians wild, and form a large part of the UK Government's justification for its current assault on doctors' professional independence. These sorts of failures form the basis for the evidence-based medicine movement that is currently so fashionable.

But seemingly irrational prescribing may have its reasons. Just as patients go to doctors for more than a biomedical fix, so medication represents far more than the biomedical screwdriver that does the fixing. Medication has a significance that goes beyond its biomedical effects; therefore, to understand it, we must again widen our gaze.

Why do patients take pills?

Have you ever had this sort of consultation? Mr Smith smilingly confirms that he takes his long-term medication regularly. The computer screen shows that you have given only three months worth of tablets over the last eight months. Mr Smith fails to see your point.

Studies repeatedly show that somewhere between 30% and 50% of prescribed medicines are not taken as directed.[11,12,13,14] Bearden et al found that 27% of young women didn't even cash in their prescriptions.[15]

Rather than bemoaning the capricious behaviour of our patients, should we not examine why compliance is so low? Isn't it time for us to focus less upon the medicine and more upon the patient? If we want to understand why patients take pills we must look beyond medicine. Our reasons for prescribing pills may come from the dramatic achievements of 20th-century pharmacology. But as often as not a patient's reasons for taking those pills stems from much older and more complex human behaviours.

The medical reasons for prescribing might be the only ones that matter to us, but remember it is the patient who makes the daily decision whether or not our pills get taken. Traditional explanations for poor compliance have tended to focus on two rather limited perspectives. One perspective sees compliance problems as evidence of a failure in doctor–patient communication.[16] Another perspective relates to health beliefs, to whether the medication fits in to the patients own belief system about his condition.[17] But perhaps we need to look back before modern therapeutics to understand the role of medication.

Homo pharmacologicus?

One of man's unique characteristics is his desire to take medicine. A 60,000-year-old burial site has been found in Iraq.[18] The body was buried with the flowers of seven plants with medicinal qualities. It seems unlikely that these medicines were taken as a result of a review of evidence from randomised controlled trials. In almost every ancient culture systems mixing magical, religious and pharmacological regimens have been practised. We cannot look at the broader significance of the drug for the patient without acknowledging that the drug has a broader significance for the doctor too.

Just as cats chase mice but don't necessarily eat them, humans chase medicines but don't necessarily take them. Obtaining medication and taking medication relate to separate drives and beliefs. They have separate rules. Pills possess many different roles in the health beliefs of the patient. Certainly the patient may share our biomedical model of his illness. If we give antibiotics for a boil or painkillers for a fracture, both the patient and we may agree what the drug is for. But there are a number of other possibilities.

The drug as an agent of control

Conrad asserts that what we categorise as compliance or non-compliance may actually be a mechanism for the patient to assert control over his disorder.

Literature review

Conrad P, 1985. The meaning of medications: another look at compliance. Social Science and Medicine; 20: 29–37.

Conrad studied 80 patients with epilepsy, and found that 34 of them (42%) varied their dose of medication from day to day according to how they felt about their illness, or how important it was for them to avoid fits on a given day. Loss of control to illness (or to doctors) is a source of anxiety and reduced self-esteem. This self-regulation was a way of reasserting a sense of control, rather than letting the illness control them.

It is not normal for an adult to slavishly follow the instructions of another unless he is compelled or strongly convinced. As James Willis points out, most of us do not follow the advice in the car owner's manual to check our tyres for stones daily.[19] We normally act on our own evaluation of the credibility of advice, and its importance to us.

In Chapter 5 we recognised that the patient has an active role in implementing coping mechanisms to get through illness. The control over taking or not taking medication is one powerful mechanism for the patients' re-assertion of their own mastery over themselves at a time when that mastery seems fragile. It is not only in ethics that we must balance beneficence with autonomy. Such a balance exists in the patients' world also.

The drug as a representation of disease

There may be a significant ambiguity in a patient's attitude to their pills. As well as representing an agent of control over the illness the pills may represent the illness itself. "If I take these pills then I am admitting I'm an epileptic." The pills are a daily memento mori of the diagnosis.

Again our internal world is programmed to offer us defences against trouble. Denial and bargaining are both effective psychologically, even as they are ineffective in terms of affecting outcome. But again the question is, whose outcome? The medical outcomes that matter are always ultimately located in someone's head. We cannot deny the validity of ego defence mechanisms as part of the total experience of coping with the threat of illness.

Where people feel an intense ambiguity they don't take a consistent middle ground, they tend to demonstrate behavioural swings. (Think about the comparison with eating disorders.) There may be no biological sense in taking antihypertensives on and off, but it is typical of normal human behaviour.

The drug as a legitimisation of the sick role.

The sick role is a social construct produced as a response to illness, with or without biomedical disease. It may excuse people from work, from washing up, even from behaving reasonably to others.[20] It must be legitimised by the doctor, whether by a prescription, a certificate, or by a prominent Tubigrip.

Quite often the sense of grievance that a patient may have if we don't prescribe for URTIs is because we appear to be failing to give official recognition to the fact they feel ill. They may feel let down, unsure as to whether they are allowed to be ill or not. A bottle of pills demonstrates that the doctor has sanctioned the illness. The pills don't have to be taken, they just have to be there.

The drug as a gift

When you are ill you need "stroking".[21] Rallying social support is an important coping mechanism. The family are supposed to give you grapes and chocolates. The doctor is supposed to give you pills.

The symbolic meaning of a gift may be much greater than its simple usefulness – who needs grapes? A prescription can be seen as an expression of care. Unfortunately, just as in the sick role, the absence of a prescription can be seen as an absence of care. Like the grapes, the pills are just as useful on the bedside table as in the stomach.

The drug acts as a "high status" gift, as it comes from an authority figure. Any friend can bring grapes, but only the doctor can bring amoxicillin. The drug may be seen as an important statement of social support, and thus be part of a social coping mechanism.

We need some way to negotiate between our world of giving pharmaco-active substances and the patients' world of the need for the trappings of medicine.

The drug as a threat

Even miracles have their downside. There are also strong negative images of medication.[22] We use the word "drug" to mean both a modern miracle pill and something that addicts inject in back alleys. Perhaps this reflects society's profound ambivalence about the whole project of science. In the media, pills are either a miracle breakthrough or the subject of a new scare. Kill or cure at the toss of an editorial coin.

Drugs are sometimes seen as "chemicals" (what isn't?), or as "unnatural" (ignoring the fact that cholera, meningitis, lighting strikes and being eaten by a shark are undesirable although eminently natural). Again this may relate to a deeper ambivalence, unease that science may be a source of wealth and security, but is at the same time a threat to our planet.

Doctors view drugs as addictive (a small minority) or non-addictive on the basis of medical evidence. The public may view drugs in general as potentially addictive. This is sometimes expressed as a reluctance to become "dependant" on a medicine, in a way that one would not express concern about the risk of becoming dependant on doorstep milk delivery or the daily paper.[23]

Cornford explores this Jeckyl and Hyde ambivalence in his qualitative study on patients' views on the use of domiciliary oxygen:

Literature review

Cornford C, 2000. Lay beliefs of patients using domiciliary oxygen: a qualitative study from general practice. British Journal of General Practice; 50: 791–3.

Cornford interviewed 24 patients receiving domiciliary oxygen therapy. Patients did not seem to use their oxygen for the defined biomedical reasons that their doctors prescribed it. For example a patient believed that "I should have had so much [oxygen] before I went out and then sort of top up again when I came back". He found a profound ambivalence in patients' beliefs in the effects of oxygen.

Like Conrad (see p. 172) he found that patients used oxygen to regain or maintain a sense of mastery. It was perceived to relieve dyspnoea, and therefore increase the patients' ability to control their daily lives by giving them a boost for particular challenges, or as a symptomatic relief if they were feeling unwell. He quotes a patient who says: "If you know it's there you seem to relax."

But Cornford also found that patients feared that using oxygen could lead to them losing mastery by coming to depend on it. He quotes a patient's view that "you have to use it in moderation. If you're going to use it all the time you're going to become dependant on it and that's something I don't want to do." So the patients perceived a risk that the drug could master them.

The drug as part of the doctor

Pills may form a cognitive link with the world of the doctor. Balint saw the doctor himself as a potent drug, and pills remind the patient of the doctor's influence in their illness behaviour.[24] Just as conscience has been thought of as an internalisation of parental influence, so the pill can be seen as an internalisation of the influence, or even the presence, of the doctor. Anthropologists have suggested that the drug can be thought of as part of the doctor being ingested into the patient, reminiscent of the host at mass.

Failure to take the pills may therefore be the equivalent of adolescent rebellion against the authority of a parent figure. Having the pills there on the mantelpiece, on the other hand, remains as necessary as having the parent still there to turn to if the worst comes to the worst.

The drug as totem

In almost every ancient culture systems mixing magical, religious and pharmacological regimens have been practised by shamans. When we are ill there is a deeply ingrained instinct to seek help from a parent figure in whom we invest a power over us. Helman points out that the modern doctor still fulfils the role of a shaman in contemporary society.[25]

Magical thinking may use objects on which we project our bargains with fate. Pellegrino observes that "the drug is the visible sign of the physician's power to heal".[26] I may invest a carefully labelled and rattling pill bottle with the same significance as a person in another time or another culture would invest in a carefully painted rattle of seed pods.

The role of shaman is socially defined, and in western societies to be a medical practitioner is a formal and legally protected status. In the UK you can only claim to be a medical practitioner if your name is on the Medical Register, established by the Medical Act of 1858. Only then can we rise from the status of friend, offering paracetamol and grapes, to that of doctor, who alone holds the power to prescribe all the wonders of the BNF. The prescription pad is therefore a badge of office both confirming and symbolising the doctor's paternalistic authority.

Prescribing is therefore part of my social role. It is my job to prescribe the medicine, and the patient's job to decide whether to take the medicine. This of course works fine for Dr Findlay prescribing Mist Gent Alk, but not so well for the 21st-century doctor prescribing the latest ACE inhibitor.

The drug as placebo

Placebo-controlled trials have repeatedly tended to show a placebo response of around 30%. In such a trial, if the active agent has a response of 31% and the trial is large enough to demonstrate that this is a significant difference, then we conclude that the active agent works.

This is an example of the medical gaze at work. We choose to concentrate on a 1% effect that fits in with our biomedical model rather than a 30% effect that we don't really understand. Why placebos work is a matter of fierce debate, and there are likely to be different mechanisms in different situations. They illustrate that the mind and body are not separate – man is not a dualistic being but a unity. Our perception of our health state can be proven in many different situations to affect our "actual" measurable health.

Book review

Dixon M and Sweeney K, 2000. The human effect in medicine. Oxford: Radcliffe Medical Press.

The authors state: "Our intention is to challenge the dogma of modern technological medicine that ignores both the therapeutic effect of the doctor and the self-healing powers of the patient."

The book gives a historical account of the conflict between the doctor as healer and as scientist, and the erosion of individual care within medicine. It "raises the question of whether we should endlessly fight disease by throwing technology at it, especially when we are unable to deliver that technology without frustrating and stressful delays".

The authors examine the placebo effect, and survey the evidence for the different mechanisms within the body and mind that may be involved. They ask whether the doctor as a physician healer could not harness these same mechanisms. The last section describes ways in which doctors could practise in a more holistic way. This would enable patients to become active self healers rather than passive consumers of medical care.

Prescribing with a wider gaze?

Option 1 – denial

Treatment guidelines agreed by expert specialist groups are usually based on biomedical evidence only. Problems with treatment tend to be recognised only within that same framework. We'll know that medicine really has a multidimensional gaze when we see "possible stigma and loss of self efficacy" listed among the side effects in the data sheet.

We criticise patients for having poor compliance with medication when sometimes the reason is their denial. But we use denial ourselves as a way of keeping medicine clear-cut when it is not.

Option 2 – inclusion

The "compliance" model sees patients not taking the medication we prescribe as a problem of patients not doing what they are told. The compliance model therefore looks for ways in which to increase the probability of patients doing as they are told, and there are plenty of research findings relevant to this.[27,28,29]

The problem with this model is that it views the patient as a passive recipient of the doctor's ideas. It portrays the patient as a rather dim child who has to be repeatedly coerced until the message finally gets through. Yet patients do not fail to take medicines because they are dim, but because they have their own models and their own priorities.

Health beliefs have roots and connections with the broader range of personal and socially related ideas that make up each individual's world. It is naive for us to think that we can simply overwrite our patients' health beliefs with our own. Respecting and exploring a patient's health beliefs is an essential part of our respect for autonomy. Why should a patient simply follow doctor's orders? Patients come to us as experts to seek our advice, but, as Tuckett pointed out, they too are experts.[30] Each patient is an expert in the experience and priorities of their own lives. Each patient is an expert in their own system of health beliefs.

So what about compliance?

In the traditional medical model of compliance with medication, it is the doctor who balances the biomedical factors and comes to a decision. The patient's task is to accept this and do as he is told. This is represented below:

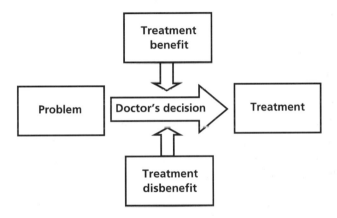

As we know that patients are not passive (and do not do as they are told) it is smarter to incorporate their evaluation of the problem and the benefits and disbenefits of a particular treatment within the consultation. The approach to the consultation advocated by Tuckett can be represented as:

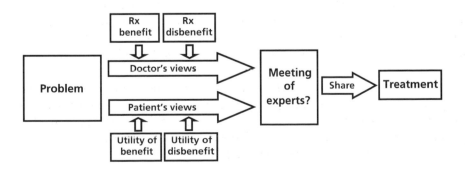

Thus the issue is not one of compliance (will the patient do what I tell him?), but of concordance (have I understood the patient's health beliefs and negotiated a course of action that both of us are happy with?).

Implications for the consultation

- Explore the patient's health beliefs. It may be relevant to find out their origin.
- Recognise that these beliefs have value – they have enabled the patient to understand and deal with their problem up to now. Whilst they could be analysed as "right" or "wrong" according to current medical orthodoxy, this is of little help to the patient.
- Compare the patient's beliefs with our own. We are likely to find both differing and shared beliefs. It may be that differing beliefs do not matter. It is better to be pragmatic.
- Recognise and value the cultural context of the patient's health beliefs.
- If differing beliefs do matter then the nature of our task is not so much "conversion to orthodoxy", but rather to build a bridge across which we can share the most important ideas and plans. This involves respecting the integrity of both models and "talking up" any shared beliefs. We can restructure what we say so that new ideas add to or modify (rather than replace) the patient's existing health belief framework.
- Consider the possible non-medical reasons for the patient wanting or not wanting to receive a scrip. How does this change the picture?
- Occasionally there is no shared ground, or it may be inadequate. We must acknowledge this and deal with the dilemma honestly.

We know that the compliance model is paternalistic and does not work. Concordance in treatment decisions cannot always be achieved, but it should be our aim. We still have to remember that many of the reasons for wanting pills are reasons to obtain a scrip rather than to take a drug. Concordance is not a panacea for problems of compliance. Concordance is, however, a step towards a more adult partnership with patients.

Remember that concordance is only a meaningful model if its outcome is allowed to differ from the compliance model. It is not a sneaky way of getting patients to do what we want. It is a way of negotiating between two different but valid perspectives, accepting that the patient makes the ultimate treatment decision.

A challenging case

Case report

Maria is a 22-year-old temporary resident from Southern Europe, who has just started working as an au pair. She attends surgery for the first time, clutching a box of metoclopramide IM ampoules. She is suffering from menorrhagia, and asks me to administer her IM metoclopramide, as this is her usual treatment and she feels it gives her relief. It has been prescribed by her own doctor from home, and is normally administered by her mother, a retired nurse.

Metoclopramide is an anti-emetic. It is not indicated for dysmenorrhoea, although it would help any associated nausea, and might possibly marginally help the absorption of analgesics. I have never heard of any doctor in the UK giving metoclopramide injections as a main treatment for dysmenorrhoea. So what are the issues I must face as I consider Maria's request to me?

Issue 1: The patient's health beliefs

Certainly dysmenorrhoea demonstrates that any simplistic model such as:

Condition A – not serious ⇒ no action
Condition B – serious ⇒ see a doctor

is inadequate if not downright fallacious. On the one hand dysmenorrhoea is painful, distressing, biological and interferes with life. Thus is may be construed as the province of the doctor. On the other hand, dysmenorrhoea is "natural", a common experience of women, not "serious", and normally treatable with OTC medication, thus it may be construed as not appropriate to take to a doctor. One could propose dysmenorrhoea as an ideal condition for demonstrating action being based on health beliefs, not biology.

Patients take action rationally on their health beliefs. Maria's actions may be influenced by:

- Her perception of the seriousness of the condition.
- Cues to act – in this case these have been reinforced by her mother, constructing the injection of metoclopramide as a normative response to dysmenorrhoea. Other cues to act may include a symptom disrupting normal life, or scare stories in the media, horror stories from a neighbour.
- What will happen if it is not treated? Fear or uncertainty re prognosis.

Health beliefs are likely to be culturally determined. In some cultures injections are seen as inherently potent and therefore desirable, irrespective of pharmacology.

Another factor that will affect how patients act on their health beliefs is their locus of control – that is to say their predominant belief about what/who will determine the outcome when a problem arises in their life.

It seems likely that Maria's LOC is projected onto powerful others. "My life in their hands." It may well be that Maria has an exaggerated faith in doctors fuelled by this LOC position. It therefore becomes the doctor's responsibility to "fix" any problem – the patient's only responsibility is to seek treatment.

It may be that this unhealthy dependence on placebo injections has been actively fostered by a system that projects the LOC onto doctors to a greater extent than is fostered by UK medicine.

Issue 2: The role of the drug

The drug may have a placebo effect

Placebos relate, in part, to the power of suggestion. The more powerful the suggestion the more powerful the effect. An injection is commonly viewed as a "powerful" intervention. The Southern European doctor may have (consciously or unconsciously) found by trial and error a powerful yet relatively harmless placebo for Maria.

The drug is a gift

Remember that Balint views the doctor himself as a powerful drug. The doctor may be seen by some as a powerful authority figure, well placed to make effective "suggestions" that may alter a patient's thoughts and beliefs about their condition. The doctor is in the socially defined role of "Shaman", having a "magical" effect over the patient and their illness.

Any gift is a significant transaction that may have a strong symbolic meaning. Thus when we give a prescription (or injection) to Maria this may have two effects:

- As a "positive stroke" showing that the doctor cares, and his protective presence is given. The human touch will be more important in this situation as Maria is ill in a foreign country, away from her family, thus making the social role of the doctor more poignant and sought after. For the doctor to deny this gift could be failing to give this support. If he wants to modify Maria's expectations he would certainly be wise to offer some equivalent gift instead, such as a prescription reinforced by careful explanation, suggestion, "positive strokes" and good rapport.
- As a symbolic ritual act, like the rattling of bones over a patient from a witch doctor, having a magical effect over the illness. Again the perceived potency of an injection will reinforce both of these effects.

The drug legitimises the sick role

This could be a crucial element in this situation – Maria is a newly arrived au pair – she is young, perhaps intimidated by the sudden change of circumstances and surroundings, perhaps anxious about her ability to carry out her responsibilities.

The sick role offers Maria a brief, socially-sanctioned escape from her responsibilities. The sick role, except in minor illness with minor escape from responsibility, must be sanctioned – authenticated – by a doctor. This is done not by a statement from the doctor (although an FM3 certificate is called a "Doctor's Statement") but by implication from the doctor's attitude and actions. Any action offering investigation or treatment implies a sanctioning of the sick role. Thus a prescription (or injection) or a referral are potent legitimisers of the sick role. Maybe Maria needs a couple of days of time out to adjust.

Issue 3: the profession of medicine

Most cases of dysmenorrhoea are successfully self treated by OTC analgesics or NSAIDs. That Maria has been carefully trained to come to a doctor seeking a powerful placebo is a clear case of medicalisation of her normal life. The medical profession has produced this response by constructing Maria's normal life as a medical problem.

This particular situation highlights the conflicts between different group norms in different medical cultures, even within Europe. Medicalisation has shot itself in the foot. Medicine is revealed as a sham if the same problem meets a completely different response in two different countries. This demonstrates that the doctor's response is determined not by biological necessity, but as group norms that have evolved for the benefit of doctors.

One can see the influence of financial incentives on these group norms. The Southern European doctor is likely to be paid under some form of fee-for-service system (whether state or private). This encourages him to prescribe potent placebos requiring medical intervention and generating income. The UK doctor is paid for having Maria on his list, but he doesn't actually want to see her! He will send her away with a prescription or advice. He will get paid as much even if she doesn't attend. To this extent the UK system could be said to limit the danger of medicalisation when compared to fee-for-service systems.

How should the UK doctor explain this conflict of practice? If he implies that the UK way is "better" or the injections in Southern Europe are unnecessary he risks damaging the monolithic mystique of the medical establishment – his own professional power base. Diplomacy will be used – whether one calls it professional etiquette or professional conspiracy depends only on one's perspective.

One might be tempted to say "Well, for goodness sake, doesn't anyone know what the optimum treatment for dysmenorrhoea is?" I know the variety of treatment options I choose from. I know what our local gynaecologists do. Or if I don't fancy that, I send the patient to a gynaecologist in the other direction who will do something different.

But there's a funny thing here. On the one hand this case demonstrates the lack of rationality of different doctor's responses, providing a strong supportive argument for an injection of EBM, not metoclopramide, into the whole situation. But on the other hand the evidence so far has demonstrated the "the problem" is not primarily a biomedical problem, but a psycho-socio-anthropological problem determined by its cultural roots and setting. If this is true it matters little whether I inject metoclopramide or phlogiston – as long as I do no harm, keep costs down and make some attempt to reach for reverse gear on the medicalisation front. So EBM will not answer the questions that face me in this consultation.

Case report: conclusions

The problem is presented in the form of two dichotomies for the doctor:

> UK doctor's management (right) versus patient's expectation (wrong).
> UK doctor's management (right) versus Southern European doctor (oh dear, oh dear).

I would wish to propose a different model of decision-making, which, apart from the ownership of the symptom, is common to all three players:

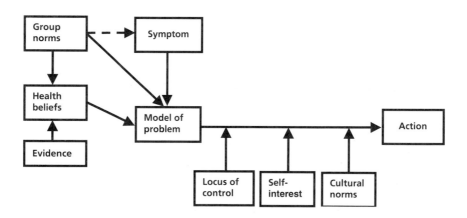

Being a doctor does not change the nature of my thought processes. It influences what is in the boxes, e.g. my health beliefs. But in fact I share a common problem-solving mechanism with my patients. So what is in these boxes that is different between doctor and patient?

Health beliefs:	Patient:	Learned from their own experience of life and cultural norms	

Doctor: Learned from their own experience of life and cultural norms + medical school + continuing medical education

Evidence:	Patient:	My auntie said ... My granny died of ... My newspaper said ... My internet search said ...

Doctor: My professor said ... My last patient died of ... My journal said ... My internet search said ...

Self-interest:	Patient:	Relief of symptoms Establishment of sick role Receipt of coping mechanisms

Doctor: Gratitude of patient Establishment of professional status Receipt of fee

The overall impression is one of similarity of thought processes; it's just that the thoughts that are in the boxes before the problem arrives are different.

It is worth trying to explore the content of these boxes for the doctor and for the patient when faced with cases where we find patients' expectations or behaviours hard to understand. By and large, doctors' and patients' behaviours are not irrational, just complicated.

Fantasy comment from the Southern European doctor

You English doctors are very snooty in your assumption that meto-clopramide is not an appropriate treatment for dysmenorrhoea. Let me make two comments.

First, as you have spent so much of this chapter saying the drug in the syringe is not the issue, why does it bother you so? You are so biomedical when you scratch the surface.

Second, I have known Maria a long time – I should: I delivered her. Her mother was my nurse. I listen to this family, I know what they want because I listen to them.

It's not always easy growing up. Maria has found the going tough. And for two days each month, well I think it all just "floods out of her". And so I help her. I do not stand back aloof with my nice neat British National Formulary. She has great faith in my injections, because she has great faith in me.

> She is growing up. She will not always need me and my "magic"
> injections. But now it helps her to know I will care for her and I am
> prepared to act to help her.
> "Witch Doctor"? – well, maybe. But I know what I am doing. And I know I
> am a doctor. I act. I intervene for the good of my patient. Why do you
> argue with that?

Conclusion

Prescribing is a minefield of conflicting systems and symbols. On one level doctors seek to prescribe "rationally", as defined by the biomedical model. But they must do this within communities that possess powerful psychological, social and anthropological dimensions.

Perhaps we should redefine rational prescribing as our ability to give an intelligent reason for the prescription, rather than the prescription being supported by evidence of biomedical benefit. This reason could include considerations of benefit and harm within these psychological, social and anthropological dimensions. Until we manage to broaden our gaze and integrate our practice, then private practice and alternative practitioners will continue to flourish.

References

1 O'Neill P 1999. Acute otitis media (clinical review). BMJ; 319: 833–5.
2 Glasziou P et al, 1999. Antibiotics versus placebo for acute otitis media in children. Cochrane Review. The Cochrane Library, Issue 3. Oxford: Update Software.
3 Report of the Welsh Antibiotic Study Group, 1999. BMJ; 319:1239–40.
4 Little P et al 1997. Reattendance and complications in a randomised trial of prescribing strategies for sore throat: the medicalising effect of prescribing antibiotics. BMJ; 315: 350–2.
5 Standing medical advisory committee (Department of Health), 1998. The path of least resistance. Main report. London: Department of Health.
6 Hart J, 1992. Rule of halves: Implications of under-diagnosis and dropout for future workload and prescribing costs in primary care. British Journal of General Practice; 42: 116–19.
7 Protheroe J et al, 2000. The impact of patients' preferences on the treatment of atrial fibrillation: observational study of patient based decision analysis. BMJ; 320: 1380–4.
8 Haines A, Jones R, 1994. Implementing findings of research. BMJ; 308: 1488–92.
9 Antman E et al, 1992. A comparison of the results of meta-analysis of randomised controlled trials and recommendations of clinical experts. JAMA; 268: 240–8.
10 Armstrong D et al, 1996. A study of general practitioners' reasons for changing their prescribing behaviour. BMJ; 312: 949–52.
11 Trestle J, 1988. Medical compliance as an ideology. Social Science and Medicine; 27: 1299–1308.
12 Harness R, Taylor D and Sackett D (eds) 1979. Compliance in health care. Baltimore: Johns Hopkins University Press.
13 DiMatteo M and DiNicola D, 1982. Achieving patient compliance. New York: Pergamon Press.
14 Jones J et al, 1995. Dicontinuation of and changes in treatment after start of new courses of antihypertensive drugs: a study of a United Kingdom population. BMJ; 311: 293–5.

15 Beardon P et al, 1993. Primary non-compliance with prescribed medication in primary care. BMJ; 308: 135–6.

16 Garrity T, 1981. Medical compliance and the clinician–patient relationship: a review. Social Science and Medicine; 15E: 215–22.

17 Becker M, 1976. Sociobehavioural determinants of compliance. In: Compliance with therapeutic regimes. Sackett D and Haynes R (eds). Baltimore: Johns Hopkins University Press. pp 40–50.

18 Leroi-Gourhan A, 1975. The Flowers found with Shanidar IV, a Neanderthal burial. Iraq Science; 190: 562–4.

19 Willis J, 1995. The paradox of progress. Oxford: Radcliffe Medical Press. p 31.

20 Armstrong D, 1989. An outline of sociology as applied to medicine. 3rd edn. London: Wright. p 7.

21 Berne E, 1968. The games people play. Harmondsworth: Penguin Books. p 14ff.

22 Britten N, 1996. Lay views of drugs and medicines: orthodox and unorthodox accounts. In: Williams S, Calnan M (eds). Modern medicine: lay perspectives and experiences. London: UCL Press.

23 Adams S, Pill R, Jones A 1997. Medication, chronic illness and identity: the perspective of people with asthma. Cocial Science and Medicine; 45: 189–201.

24 Balint M, 1964. The doctor, his patient and the illness. London: Pitman.

25 Helman C, 1990. Culture, health and illness. 2nd edn. London: Butterworth-Heinemann. pp 60 and 81.

26 Pellegrino E, 1976. Prescribing and drug ingestion, symbols and substances. Drug Intelligence and Clinical Pharmacy; 10: 624–30.

27 Hulka B et al, 1975. Practice characteristics and quality of primary medical care: the doctor–patient relationship. Med Care; 13: 808–20.

28 Ley P, 1989. Improving patients' understanding, recall, satisfaction and compliance. In A Broome (ed.). Health psychology. London: Chapman and Hall.

29 Haynes R, 1982. Improving patient compliance: An empirical review. In R Stuart (ed.). Adherence, compliance and generalisation in behavioural medicine. New York: Brunner/Mazel.

30 Tuckett D, Boulton M, Olson C and Williams A, 1985. Meetings between experts. London: Tavistock.

Discussion:
What is medicine's gaze and
who controls it?

*Medicine provides a powerful reminder ... of our "nature" as
bodily beings beset by illness and destined for death. Yet
medicine also reminds us it is our "nature" to be a community
that refuses to let suffering alienate us from one another.*
Stanley Hauerwas, Suffering Presence, 1986
*The facts all contribute to setting the problem, not to its
solution.*
Ludwig Wittgenstein

Chapter summary

Rapid societal change requires doctors to re-evaluate medicine and their
role within it. We are faced by four major questions. What is health? What
lies within medicine's gaze? How should we practise medicine? Who
controls medicine?

Change is here to stay

Could medicine be done differently? In Britain we have got so used to the NHS
that the last decade of un-navigated change and the promise of more rapid
change to come have unsettled many. Kealey repeats the conventional
description of the NHS as "the envy of the world" before going on to comment
that it is "an envy so envious that practically nobody has copied it".[1]

Change gives us a choice. We can either be victims of change, sitting back
passively while it is done to us. Or we can influence change, and seek to control
our own futures. Before we charge in with our own desperate and ill-thought-
out remedies, we should ask ourselves what medicine is for, and how its
objectives can reasonably be achieved. I would like to explore four questions:

- What is health?
- What lies within medicine's gaze?
- How should we practise medicine?
- Who controls medicine?

What is health?

We know what a car is. We can recognise one, we have opinions as to which sorts are best, and we are prepared to spend significant sums to keep them. But although we are prepared to spend dizzying sums on health care, no-one seems quite sure what health is.

The World Health Organisation made a bold offer. Their definition of health is "not merely the absence of disease or infirmity but a state of complete physical, mental and social well-being". As was noted in Chapter 1, this is a utopian vision that does not relate to any reasonable model of the real world.

The WHO definition should alert us to another paradox: the WHO definition seems dated. Its faith in an attainable Nirvana is touching, but not credible. It is a flagrantly modernistic statement, and, like a statue of Lenin, it appears now as the ironic icon of a bygone age. Our definition of health will be linked to the thinking of our time, and it will have a sell-by date.

Another approach to health is to see it in terms of norms. "Two legs good, one leg bad". Certainly I have no great desire to lose any limbs, but if I did could I not be healthy afterwards? Health as the attainment of biomedical norms is none the less becoming our dominant definition by default. It is the only definition that makes sense within a biomedical model, and we are seeing our profession driven increasingly down a razor-sharp but razor-narrow biomedical lane. A norm-referenced definition of health excludes issues such as self-image, self-efficacy and control, and ignores the difference between disease and illness.

So what is health care *for*? The preceding chapters have shown that however advanced our treatment of disease may be we can never banish illness. At the very least medicine must recognise and deal with both disease and illness, and the disability that may stem from either. Health care exists for the benefit of the patient. Health care must therefore include both processes and outcomes that are valid primarily in the world of the patient, not primarily in the world of the doctor.

We therefore have a dichotomy of aims for health care:

Option 1: Healthcare exists in order to maintain biomedical parameters within the normal range. Two legs, Na+ 136–145mml/l, diastolic below 90mmHg, no dyskaryotic cells seen. This involves controlling any aspects of patients' lives that threaten these normative measurements. Proper health care necessitates continuous surveillance of the population for possible biomedical abnormalities.

Option 2: Health care exists to enable patients to live the lives that they choose, as much as possible unencumbered by, or despite, disability. We will wish to reduce suffering where this is compatible with the patient's pursuit of their goals. We will wish to delay death where this is compatible with the patient's pursuit of their goals, and when the attempt does not produce undue suffering. Aspects of Option 1 will be used only when they serve these principles.

We have examined the implications of the Option 1 approach to health care. Now let us look at Option 2

Health – "the strength to be"

Deitrich Bonhoeffer was a German theologian whose opposition to Hitler led him to jail, suffering and ultimately execution. In the middle of a traumatic imprisonment he wrote what he could, work later published as "Letters and papers from prison".[2] Bonhoeffer defined health as "the strength to be".

OK, it's catchy, but what does it mean? Bonhoeffer is saying that health is the ability to pursue our life story without insurmountable obstruction from illness. Unless I am an Olympic skier I can be healthy even after the loss of a leg. If I am an Olympic skier I can regain health by seeking the courage to re-write my life script. By this measure Bonhoeffer died a healthy man.

Such a definition of health is relevant unless we wish to see the whole population deemed unhealthy as defined by a utopian biomedical gaze, and thus in need of medical intervention.

This definition does not decry the role of biomedicine. If there is anything that stands in the way of me fulfilling my life goals that can be fixed by biomedicine then this model tells me to fix it. But in reality there is so much sickness that we cannot fix, and this model gives me a more dynamic and a more patient-oriented way to seek ways round, or ways of coping with the unavoidable.

Peter Toon has developed this type of model in his RCGP occasional paper "Towards a philosophy of general practice: a study of the virtuous practitioner".[3] He contrasts what he calls the "biomechanical" and "interpretative" approaches to health care. He comments that "seeking pleasure and avoiding pain are not the highest goods". He advocates health care which both serves the patient's own life narrative and where possible contributes to the patient's understanding of their narrative.

One should not overestimate the divergence between the two models. With either model I will remove an inflamed appendix and give comfort to the bereaved. To get to either Birmingham or Bradford I may drive up the M1. But the difference will show up as we go further.

Question 1

Do we pursue a model of health that is based around the attainment and preservation of biological norms, or do we pursue a model of health that is based on the patient's ability to pursue their lives unimpeded by, or accommodating to, illness?

What lies within medicine's gaze?

We have considered Foucault's concept of the medical gaze.[4] No patient brings us a diagnosis. They bring us complaints. The medical model is a construct that we generate, not a truth "out there". From all the features which are brought into our consulting rooms, which do we choose to construct a medical model? It is as if a patient brings us Lego, Meccano and bricks and mortar. Which items we select determines the construct that we make.

The medical gaze determines the fabric of the medical model. It also imposes two constraints:

- If the gaze includes, it must also exclude. Our model cannot include everything. Part of the art of "taking" (or constructing) a history is knowing what to exclude ("I first had the pain in my leg the day after Aunty Vera's birthday – no it was Aunty Ruby's birthday, I know because it was the 57 bus I took that day, I had lost my bus pass and I met a man at the bus stop who…") We determine what part of the patient's story is to be used to form a medical construct. What then do we include, and what do we exclude as we construct our medical models?
- Second, the medical gaze, just like the retina, may include a hierarchy of priority. My gaze is determined by where I am looking, but my macular field of vision collects far more information than my peripheral vision, and hence contributes more to the model being built in my brain. Within our medical gaze not everything can be important. If it is, then nothing is important. What is more important and what is less important as we construct our medical models?

What determines our medical gaze cannot be separated from our belief about the nature of health. Or, to be more accurate, our operational belief: not necessarily the belief we pay lip service to. If we hold a biomedical model of health then we can be happy with a simple biomedical gaze. If we hold a WHO model of health, biomedical with knobs on, then our gaze is biomedical with the psychosocial dimensions bolted on, but not necessarily integral to the working of the structure, and conveniently placed in our peripheral vision.

If we truly believe in a multidimensional model of health, which includes the biomedical, social, psychological, anthropological and spiritual dimensions as genuine partners, then we are swimming against the stream. The current NHS reforms are staunchly biomedical and managerial in their gaze. Evidence-based medicine (and its sources such as the Cochrane database) are predominantly biomedical. We are in a culture that pays lip service to the needs of the patient, but ignores any attempt to catalogue or understand those needs. Patients' needs are multidimensional. Can our gaze rise to the challenge to see them?

So how can we make our gaze more patient-friendly? It is sometimes as if we live in one of those films that use black and white scenes to talk about one level of the story and colour to talk about another level. Our patients live their lives and encounter problems in glorious Technicolor. The medical model selects out the black and white image and ignores the rest. The picture makes sense, it appears complete, and is much admired by true artists. But it fails to convey as much of reality as it could. And let's face it, the public just doesn't go to see black and white movies anymore.

If we are to reduce suffering and contribute to the patient's ability to write an unencumbered life narrative then we must deal with the multidimensional realities that patients bring with them into our consulting rooms. We can only deal with this if we can see it. To see it we need to have a language for it.

How many oranges make a violin?

Cross-category judgements are tricky. Just as we have to learn the dangers of a favourite diagnosis, so too we must avoid the danger of a Procrustean approach to a multidimensional diagnosis. Procrustes was a highway robber in ancient Greek myth. He would tie his victims to a bed. If they were shorter than the bed he would stretch them. If they were longer he would cut off enough of their feet and legs to make them fit – a common diagnostic temptation. It is just as crass to miss an available physical diagnosis as it is to offer an automatic prescription to the bereaved. If we have been chopping the patients' legs off, diagnostically speaking, this doesn't mean the only alternative is to see the patient as all leg, and to stretch the leg to fit the space available. Our gaze should be dynamic, not static. It should not rest exclusively on any one dimension of our model, but should seek out relevant features of a patient's problem from all and any of the dimensions.

We saw in Chapter 5 that much of health-related behaviour is about coping rather than curing. We need to be frank that there is much that we cannot cure, and that McKeown's analysis may be dented but not dead.[5] Do we not have a role in helping patients to cope? Caring humanely is at least as important as having an effect upon intermediate outcome measures. But we are to care about what? Unless we are confined to juvenile or patronising "reassurance" then we need a gaze that matches the canvas of the patient's experience.

There is some room for encouragement. Tomlin et al found that GPs failed to fully embrace evidence-based medicine, as GP medicine "requires a broader vision and a more pragmatic approach which takes account of practitioners' concerns and is compatible with the complex nature of their work".[6] Quite.

Our restrictive gaze applies also to our research. We have concentrated on only the first one-and-a-half of Archie Cochrane's famous three questions: "Can it work? Does it work? Is it worth it?".[7,8] Our language limits our gaze. We can measure biomedical risks, but we have no measures for the broader disbenefits of medicalisation. Gaze and language develop together, and it is time we developed both.

Learning to look

Already we believe in "ideas, concerns and expectations", but what do we know of the worlds where such things grow? Can we use language to construct and make sense of these worlds? If we believe in a multicolour world then we need to have colour film in the camera. Again the metaphor of gaze helps us. A baby has the hard-wired equipment to see, but none the less has to learn to interpret the images that fall on the retina. A baby cannot see a 57 bus, a baby can only see a big red shape of indeterminate significance. If we have no understanding, no model, no language for a patient's anthropological needs, we will never see a patient with such a need. We will therefore conclude that there are no such needs.

Question 2

What is to be included in the medical gaze? Is it to be restricted to the biomedical, or will we adopt a multidimensional gaze? If we wish to adopt such a gaze how will we do it? Will we learn the language of these other dimensions in order to see what lies within them?

How should we practise medicine?

Clearly this builds on our answers to Questions 1 and 2. Our understanding of health and our belief as to what is legitimate to include within a multidimensional medical model are the foundations for what sort of doctors we should be. I would offer a number of opinions about how we should practise:

We should practise a "people's medicine"

Yes, I mean that we should be patient-oriented (who doesn't). But we need some model of what this means. It certainly means that our gaze should be multidimensional, and should focus on the patient's narrative, not ours. We should be prepared to deal with any of the dimensions discussed in Chapters 4 to 9, acknowledging we will not be able to meet all the patient's needs and may refer to a broad range of other agencies.

We need to respect our patients. I was reminded of this recently when a 79-year-old patient told me of his admission after a stroke. He described his long wait in A&E with the trolley sides up as being "trapped in a metal box", and commented that there should be an equivalent of the RSPCA to ensure patients are treated humanely. What a great idea! What an indictment that it should be needed. (What a contrast with our local hospice. A bed is brought down to meet the ambulance, with a hot water bottle in the bed. This is the master touch. A hot water bottle costs almost nothing, but speaks volumes about the hospice's gaze.)

Patients want doctors who will listen to them, who they can understand, and who will deal with the needs that patients bring to them. It's hardly rocket science, and yet, having had a fair amount of common sense and humanity knocked out of us by a medical education, it is a lesson that seems hard to learn.

We should resist the temptation to care for the notes or the results as a proxy for the patient. Symbols such as intermediate outcome measures are not the patient. If we value people for themselves as opposed to their symbolic role in our medical universe then we will accept their outcome measures rather than impose our own. We need to be pragmatic and choose what works for the patient rather than pursue medical purism.

The biomedical model is irredeemably modernist. Our current attempts at a bio-psycho-social model represent an improvement, a halfway house. Are we able to progress to a multidimensional model of medicine that is more at ease with the needs of a postmodern society? A medicine that offers choices, not absolutes. A medicine that is based on the patient's own evaluation of the appropriateness of these choices.

Autonomy means nothing without an understanding of the choices. Our ethics, like our medicine, has a cultural context. If we are part of a medical culture that expects patients to follow our evidence-based guidelines on a take it or leave it basis, then we are artificially restricting the patient's choice, and imposing our medical culture over the patient's legitimate model of the world.

We should include ourselves in the equation

It is easy to come to an understanding that we must treat the patient not just as a biomedical problem to be fixed. It is more challenging to accept that the implication of treating the patient as a whole person is that we as whole people enter into the equation. Who I am and how I cope with the demands of being a doctor profoundly affect what lies within the reasonable boundary of my role.

Peter Toon has explored this area in his RCGP occasional paper:

Book review

Toon P, 1999. Towards a philosophy of general practice: a study of the virtuous practitioner. London: RCGP.

Toon uses the concept of virtue in its philosophical sense. There has been a resurgence of interest in virtue as an ethical concept.[9] We have come a long way with guidelines as to how we should practice medicine. But we still find ourselves facing problems, either in the form of dilemmas where no answer seems ideal, or in terms of complexity when a deterministic solution is not available.

How can we practise in a way that addresses the real human needs of our patients in a world we can neither fully understand nor control? Toon asserts that "our view of reality is constructed not observed". He contrasts the biomechanical and the humanistic models of human selfhood, and shows that the presuppositions we take away from these competing models affect how we practise medicine. He examines issues of meaning and of responsibility.

Toon argues that ultimately we can only practise good medicine if we ourselves are in the frame. To face these sorts of challenges we need to examine the values and the personal skills of the practitioner him/herself. This does not mean the doctor has to be a perfect person. It does mean that the doctor has a need to reflect on their practice, and explore the link between their personal and professional development. It means that there is an expectation that the doctor should practise as best he can virtues such as courage, wisdom, hope and justice.

Toon is making an important statement. He is saying it is not enough to look at what we do. The world is too complex for that. We must look also at the way we do what we do, and at why we do it. And that these things are inextricably intertwined with who we are. It's the traditional educational model of "knowledge, skills and attitudes", spelt out in capital letters.

We live in times when the "what" of we do is becoming the overriding concern, as it is the only one of the four variables that can be measured. And if we were not able to measure it, we would have to trust people – which would be against the political tide.

What about personal care?

From a conference entitled "Core values for the medical profession in the 21st century" the great and the good of our profession stated as their first core value "the patient/doctor relationship should be a partnership of mutual trust, with the personal consultation remaining the bedrock of medical practice. This will be so despite the rapidly changing context, content and nature of medical practice..."[10] This value is increasingly under threat. Horder states "Erosion of the tradition of personal care is now a real danger, and its preservation is one of the great challenges we face in these times of uncertainty and confusion over the future direction of the NHS..."[11]

Others find this view outdated. I was both shocked and mesmerised by the brilliantly expounded view of Professor Colin Carnall, a management academic, speaking at our local Regional Education Conference. His view is that "the doctor/patient relationship is now transactional, not relational. The more sophisticated client will seek value, not relationship."[12] He maintained that Western medicine had changed from a personal service into a factory service, and that this was now becoming a virtual network. The emphasis is on getting the right service at the right time, not on who would provide that service.

So who is right? Haslam points out that "decisions about these matters are made for political reasons. Most decision makers are healthy. It is when people are unwell and vulnerable that they seek the doctors that they trust."[13] If we believe that we ourselves are in the frame, if we believe in personal care and if we believe in the virtuous practitioner, then we are swimming against the political tide. But at the same time we are re-affirming our identity as purposeful professionals.[14]

Question 3

How should we practise medicine? Who owns medicine's goals, what is the doctor's role in society, and how does the doctor as a person fit into the equation?

Who should control medicine?

Presumably doctor, patient and politician will say in unison: "I should". There is little doubt that in the past doctors controlled medicine, and that we still retain much control. But just as we were negotiating with the patient about a more equal share, the politicians have cut in to snatch control for themselves.

The medical profession in the UK is being controlled in ways never before imagined. Central government sets us targets for coverage of cervical smears and vaccinations. Like all markets this creates winners and losers, but we are supposed at the same time to resist acting in a market-led way by throwing refusers off the list or just moving somewhere nicer. The National Institute for Clinical Excellence (NICE) has been established by the government to assess not just individual treatments but guidelines for the management of patients, in the confident assumption that one size fits all. These guidelines are to be imposed by National Service Frameworks, and policed at a local level by new systems of clinical governance, the Commission for Health Improvement (CHI) and by regular re-accreditation. And if this is not enough then the new wider remit of the General Medical Council (GMC) will be there to encourage the stragglers.

Many of these components in themselves may be of benefit. Clearly the GMC needed overhauling if it was to live up to its aim of "guiding doctors, protecting patients". I would welcome NICE if it were a medical version of the Consumers' Association, producing a consensus journal entitled "Which Treatment?", but it is clearly more invasive in its aims.[15] And in our increasingly complex world it is appropriate for doctors to have clear mechanisms of accountability. But accountability is different from control.

What worries me is the edifice that is appearing from all these measures together. Control systems are generally used to control. When the Consumers' Association starts to police your purchasing of white goods then you know something's wrong.

Clinical judgement

Charlton points out that "throughout medicine judgement is being denigrated and replaced, despite the fact that the educated and expert judgement of a single person is often the best possible option".[16] "Clinical judgement" can be sneered at as a cover for second-rate medicine, but this is to throw the baby out with the bathwater. The human mind is designed to seek and refine best-buy solutions to complex multifactoral problems that contain significant elements of uncertainty. Atkinson and Claxton (in their wonderfully subtitled book *The Intuitive Practitioner – on the value of not always knowing what one is doing*) show how large parts of the process are subconscious.[17] If this sounds to you like mysticism, then remember the number of neurones in a human brain (Chapter 2) and compare that with the number of pathways in the average management algorithm.

Downie and Macnaughton have made a contribution to this debate which I would recommend:

Literature review

Downie R and Macnaughton J, 2000. Clinical judgement, evidence In practice. Oxford: Oxford University Press.

Downie and Macnaughton argue that clinical judgement needs to be a product of both scientific evidence and a humane attitude. It is the synthesis of a technical judgement with a humane judgement. They examine the nature and scope of scientific evidence, pointing out that the different sorts of methodology used in research often require cross-category judgements that are ultimately subjective. "Judgement is an essential part of the scientist's activities." Qualitative research techniques are compared to methods used in other disciplines such as literary criticism.

The doctor is inevitably involved in interpreting the patient's world and the scientific evidence, and their relationship to one another. The good doctor should therefore not only be trained but "broadly educated ... adaptable, being developed as a rounded person, and having a broad perspective".

Downie and Macnaughton challenge us to combine science with humanity, and apply the outcome to the unique circumstances of the individual patient. They challenge us to put a new and high value on our role as experts in cross-category judgements.

So what of those who lessen clinical judgement and replace it with central control? What is wrong with central control is very simple to answer. It supposes that we have a complete picture of the world. And it supposes that the important part of a clinical picture is biomedical. Therefore one size fits almost all. I would argue that our biomedical knowledge should be used to serve our patients' individual life plans. And as patients are people, one size fits few, and all sizes need to be freely available. I am not asking that we should be free to practise second-class medicine, but I am hoping we will remain free to practise a medicine that serves the patient, not the system.

The eternal triangle

There will always be a tension between the interests of doctors, patients and politicians. From today's perspective doctors used to hold more power than is healthy, and it is good to renegotiate our balance of power with patients.

We should accept that we are motivated by a desire to retain our power over our own profession, even as I hope we seek to hand back our past power over patients. But is it right for our own power of self-determination to be seized by politicians and managers? Where is the evidence that politicians are more trustworthy or more altruistic than doctors? Where is the evidence that managers give the public a better deal than doctors? Which professional group do the public themselves rate trustworthy? If we believe in evidence-based medicine, then let the politicians show us the evidence base for this. Charlton warns: "In the end we will simply have swapped medical self interest, which was bad enough, for managerial self interest, which is worse."[18]

Question 4

Who will win in the struggle for power between doctor, patient and politician? What evidence do we have to support the current claim of politicians to be the legitimate masters of medicine?

Conclusions

The biomedical model is irredeemably modernist. Our current attempts at a bio-psycho-social model represent an improvement, a halfway house. We should progress to a multidimensional model of medicine that is more relevant to the needs of a postmodern society. A medicine that offers choices, not absolutes. A medicine that is based on the patient's own evaluation of the appropriateness of these choices.

We need to rediscover what it is to be a healer. One can think of the doctor's role as having four components:

Biomedical technician: yes, we do fix things, and are right to be proud that we can. We are fixers who should understand the use, limits and dangers of medicine.

Shaman: a culturally-defined secular priest. A parental figure that alleviates the stress of illness and sanctions changes in the patient's social roles during illness. In Dunstan's words, we are society's "accredited moral agents".[19]

Sickness guide: an advisor/client relationship, steering people towards other services that may fix them, or facilitating coping mechanisms that will help them to maximise their "strength to be" whilst enduring illness. We translate between the patient's world and the medical world.

Witness: one who is prepared to support and listen to cathartic discharge of anxiety, and to be a witness to the darker chapters of other people's life narratives.[20] We are the naturalists of the streets and homes of our fragmented society. We listen and understand, we categorise, we try to put into words what we see. We try to help the patient continue their life narrative.

To reupholster Osler's aphorism, the doctor's role is to parent rarely, fix sometimes, translate often and listen always.

The continuous evolutionary struggle for control of medicine is in a pivotal phase. How shall we define medicine's future gaze? Who is to control the practice of medicine?

References

1 Kealey T, 2000. Foreword. In Green D and Casper L (eds). Delay, denial and dilution: the impact of NHS rationing on heart disease and cancer. London: Institute of Economic Affairs.

2 Bonhoeffer D, 1953. Letters and papers from prison. London: SCM Press.

3 Toon P, 1999. Towards a philosophy of general practice: a study of the virtuous practitioner. RCGP occasional paper number 78. London, Royal College of General Practitioners.

4 Foucault M, 1963. The birth of the clinic. Paris: Presses Universitaires de France. Translation (1989): Sheridan A. London: Routledge.

5 McKeown T, 1976. The modern rise of population. London: Edward Arnold. Chap 5: The medical contribution.

6 Tomlin Z et al, 1999. General practitioners' perceptions of effective health care. BMJ; 318: 1532–5.

7 Cochrane A, 1972. Effectiveness and efficiency: random reflections on health services. London: Nuffield Provincial Hospitals Trust.

8 Haynes B 1999. Can it work? Does it work? Is it worth it? BMJ; 319: 652–3.

9 MacIntyre A, 1985. After virtue. 2nd edn. London: Duckworth.

10 Core values for the medical profession in the 21st century. Conference report. London: British Medical Association, 1994.

11 Horder J, 1998. Conclusion. In Loudon I et al (eds). General practice under the National Health Service 1948–1997. London: Clarendon Press.

12 Carnall C, 2000. Survive or thrive! Agendas for general practice. Regional Postgraduate General Practice educational conference, South Thames (East), Guy's Hospital, 17th February.

13 Haslam D, 1999. Personal view: The beginning of the end. BMJ; 318: 1633.

14 Pelegrino E and Thomasma D, 1994. The virtues in medical practice. Oxford: Oxford University Press.

15 Miles A, Hampton J and Hurwitz B (eds), 1999. NICE, CHI and the NHS reforms, enabling excellence or imposing control? London: British Medical Association.

16 Charlton B, 1993. Personal View. Underlying trends in the health service: a master theory. BMJ; 306: 526.

17 Atkinson T and Claxton G (eds), 2000. The intuitive practitioner. Buckingham: Open

University Press. Chap 2.

18 Charlton B, 1993. Personal View. Underlying trends in the health service: a master theory. BMJ; 306: 526.

19 Dunstan G, 1994. The John Hunt Lecture, 8 September. Royal College of General Practitioners.

20 Heath I, 1995. The mystery of general practice. London: The Nuffield Trust.

Index